The
Living Medicine

Also by Lina Zeldovich

*The Other Dark Matter: The Science and
Business of Turning Waste into Wealth and Health*

The
Living Medicine

How a Lifesaving Cure
Was Nearly Lost—and Why It Will
Rescue Us When Antibiotics Fail

Lina Zeldovich

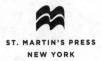

ST. MARTIN'S PRESS
NEW YORK

First published in the United States by St. Martin's Press,
an imprint of St. Martin's Publishing Group

THE LIVING MEDICINE. Copyright © 2024 by Lina Zeldovich. All rights reserved.
Printed in the United States of America. For information, address St. Martin's
Publishing Group, 120 Broadway, New York, NY 10271.

www.stmartins.com

Designed by Susan Walsh

The Library of Congress Cataloging-in-Publication Data
is available upon request.

ISBN 978-1-250-28338-2 (hardcover)
ISBN 978-1-250-28339-9 (ebook)

Our books may be purchased in bulk for promotional, educational, or business
use. Please contact your local bookseller or the Macmillan Corporate and
Premium Sales Department at 1-800-221-7945, extension 5442, or by email
at MacmillanSpecialMarkets@macmillan.com.

First Edition: 2024

10   9   8   7   6   5   4   3   2   1

*To my parents, whose courage to dissent
in the dictatorial Soviet state taught me to never give up.
To my husband and children,
who always believe in me, my passions, and my dreams.*

CONTENTS

AUTHOR'S NOTE

I don't remember when I first saw the word *phage*, but it was shortly after I learned to read in Russian, my native language. As a child, I was fascinated by how letters were drawn and how they formed words. In Cyrillic, some letters looked like skinny stick figures, some like round balloons, and others like humans standing in funny positions. In Russian, the word *phage* is spelled ФАГ, where the Ф accounts for the *f* sound. What drew my attention to the word ФАГ was the illustration—the phage figure depicted on the magazine's page looked a bit like the letter Ф itself. To my five-year-old eyes, the ФАГ figurine looked like a tough, self-confident person with its arms on the hips, radiating a clear message: *Don't mess with me!*

I came across the term inside a scientific journal that my family subscribed to. My grandmother was a chemist, my father a physicist, my mother and grandfather were engineers, so the brainy periodicals were part of my reading list. Once I learned to string letters into words, I read everything I could lay my hands on, from children's books to newspapers to medical encyclopedias. It didn't matter that I didn't understand the complex scientific topics. I read these articles not as stories but as puzzles, from which occasionally—if I managed to figure out enough words to form a sentence—I could deduce some meaning. And if not, the long, weird-looking scientific words were fun to stare at. Compared to most of them, ФАГ was so short, it almost didn't belong.

The rest of the words were much longer and more confusing, so I almost gave up on the text. But then I spotted a familiar term farther down. Дизентерия—dysentery. Not only did I know the word, I had been closely acquainted with the disease itself. The previous summer, scores of kids had fallen ill because of a contaminated grape shipment. The memories of vicious stomach cramps and endless runs to the bathroom were still vivid in my mind. My parents had fed me bowls of gooey rice cereal to quell the diarrhea—loads and loads of white slop. When that didn't help, a doctor prescribed an antibiotic, but it was sold out everywhere because so many people were sick. Finally, my grandfather traveled to the main pharmacy in the city center to bring me the coveted box.

As I read on, weaving through the long and complex sentences, I realized that this ФАГ character was actually a type of medicine that could cure dysentery. The article talked about children somewhere drinking it as a treatment. Apparently, inside your stomach, phages could kill the dysentery-causing bacteria, acting like guardians of sorts. I wondered why didn't I drink some phages? Perhaps the pharmacies didn't have it, I decided. I also decided that such a cool creature deserved more color than the magazine's dull black and white. I brought my colored pencils and retouched the phage picture with some vibrant hues.

A few years later in middle school, I stumbled upon phages again, this time in a memoir by a female Soviet scientist who had been sent to the Stalingrad front lines in World War II to ward off an impending epidemic of cholera—and avoid losing the city to the Nazis. Unlike the cryptic study I'd attempted to decipher as a kindergartener, this story read like a thriller. I understood that phages were viruses that, unlike the flu, attacked bacteria only. The idea that humans could sic these microscopic but formidable creatures onto our worst enemies seemed brilliant to me. Mother Nature, I thought, had given us these healing viruses as allies.

About a decade later, when perestroika brought down the Soviet regime and my dissident parents—banned from leaving the country for fifteen years—were finally allowed to emigrate to the

United States, we took a farewell trip to Tbilisi, the capital of Georgia. I still read anything I could lay my hands on, so in some local newspaper I picked up along the way, I spotted a familiar three-letter word—my old friend ФАГ. The article was about Tbilisi's institute that produced phages to use as medicines. At the time, my family's conversations revolved around how different our life in America would be. From freedom of speech to foods available in every store rather than rationed through endless lines, we expected our new country to be superior to the old one in every aspect of life. I could only imagine what American science was doing with phages.

Some twelve years later, when the BBC released a documentary about phage research in Georgia, I learned how naive I had been in my assumption. The documentary revealed that the Tbilisi Institute—by then renamed after its founder, Giorgi Eliava, who had been executed during Stalin's terror—was a time capsule of sorts, preserving phage wisdom for over a century while the rest of the world had long written off that treatment. I began digging up every bit of ФАГ history I could find and soon realized I was reading not just a science story but a heartbreaking human one. Over the years, I pieced that story together. From old Soviet science publications, modern-day journals, newspaper clippings, memoirs, handwritten notes, and oral histories, I re-created the narrative of the once prominent and then nearly forgotten medicine that today promises to save more lives than ever, and the incredible human beings that made it possible.

The healing viruses have been around for millions of years. They might be our best defense against the next pandemic.

The
Living Medicine

1

The Surge of the Superbugs

It may have been the slightly dirty glass you drank from at the picnic. Or it may have been the water you accidentally gulped down while swimming in the lake. Or maybe you just didn't wash your hands enough after using the public bathroom. But somehow, somewhere, you managed to swallow about a dozen hairy, rodlike germs named shigella. They slipped down your esophagus and snuggled next to your intestinal wall. Each then drew out a tiny pincer, punctured your cells, and injected them with a chemical cocktail designed to disrupt the protective outer membrane that normally keeps dangerous invaders out. Confused by the chemicals, your cells opened up and let shigella in, where it quickly set to work, chewing up your insides.

Unlike many other bacteria, shigella can't move or swim on its own, because it lacks propelling filaments. So it overtakes a cell's transporting equipment normally used to shuttle around nutrients. It hijacks the proteins floating within the cell and assembles them into so-called comet tails, which act like mini-rockets propelling shigella around—and into other cells. After shigella grows and multiplies inside the cells it invades, it kills them, moving onto its next victims. Along the way, shigella spits out a toxin that damages blood vessels, making you bleed inside. You may not feel your cells bleeding and dying during those early moments of shigella-induced dysentery, but your stomach already begins to churn.[1]

When your next bout of diarrhea turns bloody, you rush to the doctor's office. The doctor starts you on azithromycin, an antibiotic commonly prescribed for intestinal infections like the garden-variety stomach bug.[2] The problem is that the particular shigella you picked up isn't a garden variety. This shigella is tough. Its ancestors have stood up to a slew of different antibiotics, and while they saw scores of their relatives die, they were the ones that lived. They are very well equipped to combat your antibiotic weaponry.

You take your first dose and the second one, hoping for quick relief. But that's not what happens. Shigella has already detected the antibiotic molecules, so its genetic defenses are feverishly chugging out a special enzyme that slices azithromycin like a pair of scissors. Three days later, exhausted and worried, you're back to the doctor. You leave with a prescription for ciprofloxacin or Cipro, a stronger, broad-range antibiotic that should kill everything in its path, including your own, beneficial intestinal microorganisms. It may damage your microbiome, but you have no choice. You leave relieved, sure that the end is in sight.

Two days later, dehydrated, with your fever spiking, your heart racing, and your blood pressure plummeting, you wind up in a hospital, hooked up to an IV. The toxin that damaged your gut blood vessels snuck into your bloodstream, sending you into kidney failure.[3] As doctors urgently run tests, they finally discover that the vicious bacterial infection that is poisoning your insides is the broadly drug-resistant XDR shigella.[4] Because this bacteria is so new, the Centers for Disease Control and Prevention (CDC) doesn't yet offer guidelines on how to treat it, but the risk is well known; in February 2023, the CDC hosted a webinar[5] to alert doctors of its dangers. The hospital's infectious disease specialist starts you on colistin, the antibiotic of last resort, which doctors use only when all else fails because of its long list of side effects, from chest pains to numbness. But you're heading into kidney failure, so it's a question of life and death. Either you or the bug has to go.

Unfortunately, this shigella has more genetic tricks up its hairy sleeve, or rather inside its DNA. It finds a way to dodge colistin too. As it multiplies inside you, it shifts the structure of its outer cell membrane ever so slightly—just enough to make it impervious to colistin, because the medicine can no longer cling to the germ and destroy it. It's as if the bug wraps itself into an invisibility cloak. You may feel better while colistin initially kills all the vulnerable shigella, but they're soon replaced by a population the antibiotic can't destroy. Your fever spikes again, your kidneys shut down, and your heart follows, sending you into multi-organ failure.

Sadly, you're far from being an exception. Four people die every hour from an antibiotic-resistant bacterial infection in the United States.[6] That's why some scientists say that we've entered the post-antibiotic era.

It didn't have to be that way. Instead of prescribing an antibiotic, your doctors could have given you a vial of bacteriophage, a special type of virus that preys on bacteria only. With oblong bodies, spidery legs, and sharp, scorpion-like tails, bacteriophages look like miniature rocket ships from outer space. A thousand times smaller than their prey, they pierce bacteria with their tails, sneak in like Trojan horses, and burst the germs open. Bacteriophages, or phages for short, don't injure any other cells or tissues in our bodies. Instead, these viruses can destroy the harmful bacteria and leave intact the beneficial ones that help us digest food or protect us from infections. They are the healing viruses, unlike Covid or Ebola or countless others that cause deadly diseases. Had you taken the shigella bacteriophage, you likely would have recovered within a few days.

Unfortunately, you can't yet buy a bottle of bacteriophage in your local pharmacy—not over the counter or by prescription. They are not available as medications yet, at all. But in the era of skyrocketing antibiotic resistance, these phages might be our best weapons against the next bacterial pandemics.

"Phages can be powerful allies in our rapidly escalating super-bug fight," says Alexander "Sandro" Sulakvelidze, a microbiologist and founder of Intralytix, a biotechnology company that makes shigella-killing phages for a newly launched clinical trial. "Phages have been preying on bacteria for millions of years before humans came along. They are very good at it."[7] They are also constantly evolving, just like bacteria themselves. That's why it's much harder for bacteria to develop resistance to a phage than to an antibiotic. The bacteria will mutate to evade a phage, but the phages will quickly catch up and evolve to attack the bugs more effectively. Recent one-off experimental phage treatments for antibiotic-resistant infections proved to be near-miraculous cures, sometimes bringing patients back from the brink of death.

Humans desperately need these alternatives. The deaths from antibiotic-resistant infections are climbing dramatically. First commercially produced in the 1940s, antibiotics were called wonder drugs for their ability to cure almost anything. Early on, penicillin, amoxicillin, and their tougher cousin methicillin snuffed out most bacterial infections. Yet the germs soon evolved to dodge our magic bullets. Humans responded by designing stronger and more expensive armor—ciprofloxacin, gentamicin, vancomycin—but then the bugs bolstered their defenses too. A common *Staphylococcus aureus*, or staph, that once succumbed to wonder drugs can now shrug them off. Today, this stubborn staph strain has its own name: methicillin-resistant *Staphylococcus aureus*, or MRSA. This dreaded superbug now lurks in hospitals, sickening nearly 120,000 Americans per year and killing about 20,000.[8] It currently responds to vancomycin but might learn to repel it. A vancomycin-resistant enterococcus, or VRE, kills about 1 in 10 people it infects.[9] Certain strains of *Clostridioides difficile* sicken almost 224,000 Americans each year, and also dodge vancomycin, killing at least 12,800.[10] A study published in *The Lancet* attributed 1.27 million deaths to antimicrobial resistance in 2019 alone.[11]

Covid made things worse. It wiped out years of progress in our antibacterial war, says CDC's 2022 special report *COVID-19: U.S. Impact on Antimicrobial Resistance*. The coronavirus weakened patients' immune systems so that they could no longer fight off even garden-variety germs. Doctors had no choice but to prescribe more and more antibiotics. The increased antibiotic use led to a 15 percent spike in various resistant infections in 2020 alone. MRSA and VRE cases grew by 13 and 14 percent, respectively. Two other scourges, *Pseudomonas aeruginosa* and Enterobacterales, found in hospitals and often resistant to multiple antibiotics, spiked over 30 percent.

The CDC's report warns that antimicrobial resistance is already a leading cause of death globally,[12] but the future looks even grimmer. If we don't find better alternatives to our quickly diminishing antibiotic arsenal by 2050, the deadly toll of bacterial disease can reach ten million annually,[13] according to the United Nations estimate. That far surpasses the number of lives Covid claimed. In addition to new diseases, we might see the return of older plagues once thought vanquished. Covid, for example, has nothing on the truly scary microbial monsters like *Yersinia pestis*, the bubonic plague that depopulated Europe in the Middle Ages. Its respiratory airborne version, called the *pneumonic plague*, kills most people who catch it. "Pneumonic plague is rare because humans don't commonly interact with rodents that carry it, but we know that hot spots exist, both in Asia and in the Unites States," Sandro explains. "And just like Covid, it takes a few days to make you sick, so you can travel and spread it far and wide.[14] An outbreak of *Y. pestis* will be far more deadly than Covid. And if it develops antibiotic resistance, we'll be in dire shape."

The growing antibiotic resistance troubled scientists even during the pandemic. With his utmost attention on the coronavirus, Anthony Fauci, then the director of the National Institute of Allergy and Infectious Diseases (NIAID), still found time to speak about this existential threat. "In recent decades, multidrug-resistant bacteria, particularly those that cause potentially deadly diseases like tuberculosis, have become a serious and growing global public health concern," Fauci said. Bacteriophages are viable alternatives, and Fauci emphasized that research is "needed to determine if phage therapy might be used in combination with antibiotics—or replace them altogether—in treating evolving antibiotic-resistant bacterial diseases."[15]

That's exactly what Intralytix is doing. The first American biotech company to get an NIAID grant to test phage medicines in humans, Intralytix is now running three clinical trials. The first, launched with the Mount Sinai Hospital before the pandemic and delayed because of it, is using phages against a specific strain of *Escherichia coli* (*E. coli*) implicated in Crohn's disease, a chronic intestinal inflammation with no cure. If phages are effective in wiping out that pathogenic *E. coli* strain that fuels Crohn's, they will prove their worth as agents that can fine-tune our microbiome, offering new ways to treat chronic digestive problems. The shigella trial, backed by a $7 million grant from the National Institutes of Health (NIH), just started recruiting patients at the University of Maryland School of Medicine. The third trial, recently approved by the Food and Drug Administration (FDA), will pit phages against VRE, the very superbug that surged during Covid.

It may sound bizarre that viruses can heal, cure, and protect against disease, but phages play a vital role in the human virome—a viral counterpart of our microbiome, which safeguards us from pathogens we encounter constantly. "Phages naturally live in and on us—in our nose, throat, skin, and gut, protecting us from harmful bacteria," Sandro says. That's why phages are sometimes called living medicines, even though scientists are still debating whether viruses are too primitive to be considered alive.

As living medicines, however, phages are very different from antibiotics.

Antibiotics are fixed, static molecules that poison bacteria. Typically, they work by breaking bacterial cells or halting their replication. The cells wither or rupture, spilling out their microbial guts and dying. But we have used antibiotics too often. Doctors overprescribe them to patients, dishing them out when they aren't necessary. We overuse them in agriculture, indiscriminately feeding them to livestock. We over-add them to cleaning products to eliminate germs from our homes. To survive, the bugs mutated their genes and learned to produce their own molecules that destroy our antibiotic ones. Some germs produce enzymes that act like molecular scissors, shredding antibiotic molecules before they have a chance to act. Other germs surround themselves in protective cloaks or eject antibiotics from their cells before they take effect. That's the unfortunate side effect of evolution. We bred our superbugs ourselves.

We used to think that we could outpace bacterial evolution with our pharmaceutical prowess, but they mutate faster than we can keep up. Pharmaceutical research can't foretell with certainty what germs will learn or how they will change when faced with a threat, so it's impossible to stay a step ahead of them. "You can't outrun Mother Nature," Sandro tells me.

Phages operate very differently. They do the guesswork for us.

Unlike the static molecules of antibiotics, phages are biological entities that fend for themselves—attacking, multiplying, and mutating like all other creatures on earth. Phages have been feeding on bacteria for eons, so they are better equipped than our pharmaceutical industry to keep up with bacterial evolution. Scientists don't have to invent a new phage if it loses grip on its prey. They just need to slosh phages and bacteria together in a test tube, let them fight each other, and harvest the winners.

Phages have other advantages too. They are highly specialized in their microbial diet. A particular phage will only kill the specific bacteria it feeds on, leaving others intact. Phages that kill shigella or salmonella will not harm acidophilus or firmicutes—our native gut bacteria, which we need for digestion and nutrient absorption. That's a big win over antibiotics that carpet-bomb our intestinal tract, wreaking havoc on our microbiome. Unlike taking antibiotics, drinking phages would destroy only the pathogenic bugs while leaving the good ones intact.

Finding phages is also significantly easier than making antibiotics. Phages are abundant in water, soil, and especially in sewage. "They are the most plentiful biological entities in any habitat, but sewage is particularly good for phage-hunting because it's teeming with various bacteria that becomes phage food," Sandro says.[16] To date, Intralytix has harvested hundreds of species of phages, most of which were fished out from sewage plants with the goal of eventually turning them into medicinal agents. Sandro's team still makes such phage-hunting trips, because not every phage will devour every bug. Intralytix specializes in identifying the right phages for the right bacteria.

In my quest to learn more about the phage therapy revival, I visited Intralytix several times over the last few years. First conceived in 1998, when Sandro was growing *Yersinia* cultures at the University of Maryland's infectious diseases lab as a postdoc who had recently arrived from the crumbling Soviet Union, his company now occupies its own building, surrounded by Maryland woods, and uses high-tech equipment to find the right phages. "Given the near-infinite number of combinations one needs to test, it's not a task a human can muster in a reasonable amount of time. It would take months, if not years. So we don't use humans anymore," Sandro says as we walk into his lab. "We use robots. Let me introduce you to Neptune."

A biotech robot the size of a living room with a price tag of $2 million, Neptune stages microbial warfare between bacteria and phages inside ninety-six-well plates. Humans set the stage: pipette in the raw sewage; load up the target bacteria; and supply some bouillon to feed the bacteria so they can grow and multiply, becoming phage food. When loaded, Neptune whirs to life, lining up seven ninety-six-well battlefields, in which it doles out precise amounts of bouillon, bugs, and phages with its automated seven-pipette arm. Finally, it whisks the plates into an incubator attached to its back, where phages will mount their attack—but not before Neptune runs the initial health check on the troops to note their starting numbers.

"It has a way of reading how many bacterial cells are floating in the solution right now," Sandro explains to me as I watch Neptune's manipulations, mesmerized by its precision and perfection. "It will do these reads every half hour to see whether bacteria are proliferating or decreasing. At first, their population will grow, but then it should drop. That's how we know we've got good phages."

To isolate phages against specific germs, for instance, to identify the most potent shigella destroyers, Neptune will preload the plates with shigella's favorite meal—a soup of glucose, amino acids, and iron, which it finds inside our gut. Then Neptune drops the same amount of shigella in every well before adding different shigella phages, or different combinations of them, into the wells. This reveals which phage will extinguish the shigella most efficiently. With that information loaded into Intralytix's Information Management System, its PhageSelector arm can whip up a remedy recipe for any number of bacterial strains it knows, and its PhagePredictor, an artificial intelligence network, can extrapolate that information for novel strains and phages to attack them.

Even a few years ago, lab technicians would pipette every-thing by hand, toiling for days. Today, the robot does the same job a thousand times faster—and without making a single mis-take. "Imagine testing one hundred different phages on one hun-dred different shigella strains, and in different concentrations. It would take a person several months to try all these combinations," Sandro says. And then he adds affectionately, like a proud father of a prodigy kid, "But Neptune does it in twenty-four to seventy-two hours! We spent a year custom-designing it, so it's one of a kind."

While plates incubate, Sandro shows me his phage factory and warehouse. In addition to doing clinical trials, Intralytix manufac-tures and sells five FDA-approved phage preparations for the food industry. The CDC estimates that every year, one in seven Amer-icans falls ill from foodborne bugs—salmonella, listeria, shigella, E. coli, or campylobacter. That tallies up to 48 million cases, with 120,000 hospitalizations and 3,000 deaths.[17] The germs slip in via contaminated lettuce, hitchhike on sausages, and sneak into burg-ers. To decontaminate our food supply, companies use harsh steril-izing chemicals, such as chlorine or peracetic acid. Intralytix offers a more holistic and natural method: phage sprays, which combat some of the most common bacteria—SalmoFresh, ListShield, ShigaShield, EcoShield, and CampyShield. The sprays kill more efficiently and selectively than chemicals. Because phages continue to multiply for as long as there are bacteria to chew on, they only stop when no germs are left—and they only wipe out the pathogenic ones, leaving beneficial microorganisms intact.

To make sprays, Intralytix grows phages inside enormous fermenters—one-thousand-liter or about 264-gallon shiny stain-less steel towers installed in a room adjacent to the lab. Inside, phages feed on their favorite bacterial fodder until their numbers grow large enough to harvest, purify, and pour into bottles. They can also be dried and shipped in powder form to be added to water later.

The plates are still incubating, so we head over to Sandro's office to play with the PhageSelector, which formulates custom-remedy recipes based on years of data collection that preceded Neptune's arrival. The login screen flashes a green letter *I*—Intralytix—that looks like a chess figurine and greets me with a spread of pathogenic names, from common listerias to rare acinetobacters. We select bacteria to target—for example, all 1,234 strains of salmonella gathered in Intralytix's database, many of which may randomly lurk in a chicken factory. The electronic brain immediately spits out a recipe: this nine-phage brew will kill 100 percent of the bacteria. Next, we ask what it would take to extinguish particular shigella strains that, for example, originated from Chile. Turns out we'd need only two phages.

PhageSelector works the same way for medicinal use. "That's how we designed our EcoActive cocktail for Crohn's patients in the Mount Sinai study," Sandro reveals, clicking through the screens. Intralytix collected the specific strains of invasive *E. coli* found in the patients' guts. Sandro would feed the strains' info into the system and have the recipe seconds later. The Intralytix team would mix the phages and ship them off to Mount Sinai.

"As soon as Neptune enters a new phage into our system, I can formulate a cocktail against that bacterial strain, whether from my office, home, or any part of the planet," he says. "And we have a few hundred well-characterized phages in our freezers. We even have phages for *Y. pestis*, which we tested in rats—and they worked great. If a request comes for particular bacterial strains, I can design that cocktail on the spot."[18] Meanwhile, PhageSelector's sister system PhagePredictor can extrapolate information from the already existing knowledge, foreseeing cocktails' efficacies for cases Neptune hasn't tried yet.

This next-generation AI method might as well be humankind's magic armor against bacterial infectious disease of the twenty-first century. It took Sandro twenty-five years to assemble and nearly as long to convince the FDA that phages were medicinally safe. Even though phages have been widely used for decades in Sandro's homeland, to the American medical establishment, they were as foreign as space aliens. He worked long and hard to change this view. When the FDA finally green-lighted the Intralytix Crohn's trial in 2018—the first such trial in the agency's history—it marked a massive mindset shift.

"Was it worth a quarter-century-long effort?" I ask.

Sandro chuckles. "Had I known how hard it would be when I first started, I might not have pursued it," he quips, assembling the next brew on his screen, this time for vaginal infections. Once grown, this cocktail will be shipped to his collaborators in Georgia for another clinical trial starting in a few weeks. "But I was so shocked that in America people died from infections we treated in Tbilisi with medicines I grew up drinking, that I just couldn't let go. As a scientist, I had no choice but to keep pushing."

LIFE WORKS IN MYSTERIOUS WAYS

Raised in Tbilisi, an ancient city dating back to the fifth century, Sandro grew up in an apartment on the same floor as his three cousins, where the kids constantly ran back and forth across the hall, leaving the doors wide open. From that six-story apartment building, Sandro walked to school, ran to meet his mother coming home from work, and rode his bike down to the neighborhood's Vake Park, buzzing underneath the crown of grapevines that formed a canopy over the road. In the distance stood the snow-peaked Caucasus Mountains.[19]

Sandro's childhood shattered at age twelve, when his mother fell ill. Though she complained of sore spots around her spine, she didn't think much of it. When she finally went to the doctor, it was too late. The tumor had spread to her bones, spine, and tissues. That night, the family gathered and called Sandro to tell him the bad news. He knew the moment he walked into the room, because he turned bright red before anyone spoke. He took it like an adult, fought back tears, and didn't cry.[20] When his mother died, Sandro's aunt stepped in to take care of him.[21]

Sandro grew up accustomed to phage medicines. In Tbilisi, they were sold in little vials at every pharmacy, next to aspirin. People drank phage remedies for stomach bugs. They gargled with them to cure sore throats. Made at Tbilisi's Institute of Bacteriophage, Microbiology, and Virology, an organization so well hidden behind the Iron Curtain that barely anyone in the West had heard of it, the remedies were part of the everyday first aid tool kit. People kept them in medicine cabinets. They packed some when they went on vacation. Founded by a luminary yet tragic early Soviet-era scientist, Giorgi Eliava, and eventually named after him, the institute sat on the banks of the Mtkvari River, from where many of the phages were sourced. The research team cultivated the phages to make medicines against the most notorious scourges—shigella, cholera, staph. They loaded phages into bottles and ampoules and shipped them to pharmacies in Georgia and other parts of the Soviet Union.

Patients battling stubborn skin, throat, ear, and gut infections flocked to the institute from across the country. The Eliava doctors took their swabs and stool samples, identified bacterial culprits, and matched them with phages that preyed on those specific strains. It was personalized medicine at its finest—decades before the term was even coined. Sometimes phages worked fast enough that patients could go home after a few days. Stubborn infections took several weeks or even months. Sometimes patients went home with a supply of ampoules. The most obstinate cases sometimes required extra research and trial and error in assembling a personalized phage mix—formulated specifically to match the bacterial strains the person carried.

Eliava researchers constantly looked for new phages, mixed different phages together, and tried these cocktails on various bacterial strains. Long before Neptune-like robots existed, they did it all by hand, painstakingly pipetting bacteria, its food, and its predators together. They recorded their results in cursive, in big books of lined paper, painstakingly filling out numbers, ratios, sizes, and dates. When they zeroed in on a cocktail that worked well against a particular malady, they added it to their arsenal of living medicines, filing it away in those cursive-filled books.

In the West, antibiotics reigned supreme ever since they were mass-produced after World War II. But the Soviet Union never quite mastered the feat due to the peculiar quirks of the country's economy and medical system. The Soviets struggled with mass production of antibiotics because that required factories, specialized equipment, and a steady supply of chemical reagents. In the USSR, known for shortages of almost everything, a factory could run out of reagents and sit idle for a month. Phages, on the contrary, were always available—and if not, could be grown.

When Sandro announced that he was going to study biology at Tbilisi State University, his father, Levan, an engineer, was not amused. Georgia's traditional gender stereotypes deemed biology a woman's profession. Men were expected to be out in the world braving nature, weathering storms, and defeating the elements. They were supposed to build bridges, erect buildings, and lay train tracks through the frozen Siberian woods. The women, as more delicate and finer creatures, were supposed to pursue gentler disciplines that kept them out of harm's way. Biology, the majority of which took place inside comfortable lab conditions, was viewed as women's work—but Sandro was not easily dissuaded.

"I was really interested in microbes and genetics, so I went against my family to pursue it," he says. "Eventually, my dad accepted the fact that I will be 'chasing butterflies' for a living and let me be." Sandro earned his PhD in microbiology and epidemiology, with a focus on molecular biology—a new discipline at the time. His dissertation advisor was the Eliava Institute's director, Teimuraz Chanishvili, and his thesis focused on identifying *Yersinia enterocolitica* by cutting the bug's DNA into the so-called bacterial fingerprints. A distant cousin of the plague-causing *Y. pestis*, *Y. enterocolitica* was far less dangerous, but still caused stomach problems, making it a worthy research subject.[22]

Sandro's cutting-edge research career moved fast. In 1990, at age twenty-seven, he was appointed a director of the molecular biology program at the Georgian Anti-plague Center, now called the National Center for Disease Control (NCDC)—the region's equivalent of the CDC—and tasked with keeping all infectious disease outbreaks under control. "Molecular biology was in its infancy in Georgia, and my job was to establish it as a discipline," he recalls. "I was the head of the lab, and I had the entire floor in NCDC with several people working for me." He was eager to pursue every opportunity in Georgia.

During the Soviet era, the Eliava Institute, back then called the Institute of Vaccines and Serums, and the newly established NCDC were prestigious and innovative. There was money for research. Scientists were well paid. Sandro's personal life was equally exciting. With a mop of curly black hair and disarming smile, he enjoyed a varied life. He became engaged to a young journalist, Nino Kasvadze, had a circle of close friends, and explored daring hobbies. He was a contestant on the Russian version of *Jeopardy!* and once almost won a car. He learned karate, a banned sport under the

Soviet regime, which only made it more enticing. He went scuba diving with his friends from the military. Despite his ambitions, he never planned to leave Tbilisi. "Back then, you were born in the same city, went to school in the same city, got your degree in the same city, worked, got married, and raised a family—all in the same place," he recalls. "I never expected to do anything else—and why would I? I had a great Soviet career."[23]

And then, the Soviet Union fell apart.

After the USSR dissolved in 1991, Georgia declared its independence—and plunged into chaos. Elected in May of 1991, President Zviad Gamsakhurdia was ousted in a military coup the following year and fled the country, while attempting to govern from exile. The fallout wreaked havoc in science.

"You couldn't get chemicals to do experiments," Sandro recalls. "You'd spend hours on the phone with Moscow and get nowhere. You'd go to Moscow and beg for the reagents you needed and you still couldn't get any." Things grew worse when Tbilisi started having power outages—now scientists couldn't stage their reactions even if they had the chemicals. There were days with no electricity, weeks with no gas, and months with no hot water. When buildings lost heat in winter, people started chopping up wood, building fires in their apartments to keep warm. Morose and forlorn, scientists came to work to play chess and dominoes, or simply stare out the windows of their vacant laboratories. Sandro felt his best years were being squandered.[24] One of his colleagues, Nina Chanishvili—then a phage researcher at the Eliava Institute—landed a yearlong fellowship in Geneva.[25] Sandro decided to look abroad too. "I felt that I was wasting my life away," he says. "I started looking elsewhere."

He applied for several postdoctoral positions in America, Europe, and Australia. Mailing the envelopes from Tbilisi's post office felt like sending them into a black hole. In 1993, mail took up to sixty days to cross the ocean, so by the time the envelope landed on someone's desk, the deadline could have passed. Yet to Sandro's delight, the American Association for the Advancement of Science granted him funding for a fellowship position. Now he had to find a research institution to take him in. He wrote to three different places and waited.[26]

The most interesting offer came from well-known infectious disease expert Glenn Morris at the University of Maryland. Morris studied *Yersinia* and wanted to compare the disease-causing mechanisms of different strains. "I had never worked with anyone from Georgia, so I thought it was worth a try," Morris says. He wrote Sandro an offer for a nine-month postdoctoral fellowship.

Replying to Morris was an endeavor. Time was tight, so Sandro couldn't answer by mail. "I had to find a fax machine because my institute didn't have one," he remembers. "Good luck finding one in Tbilisi when electricity cuts out." But the fax was sent, and Morris helped too. He fixed some mistakes on Sandro's application, filled out some boxes he missed, and pushed the papers through. Sandro's NCDC director promised to keep his position open until he came back home next year, with more knowledge and expertise. Sandro wanted to bring his fiancée along, but the meager fellowship of $12,000 wouldn't cover living expenses and airplane tickets for two. The couple decided Sandro would go alone. Nine months would pass quickly—he'd be back home by spring. By then, the political situation would improve, electricity would return, and doing research would be possible again. Or so they hoped.[27]

In early fall, Sandro packed a suitcase, hugged his dad, aunts, uncles, and cousins, kissed his fiancée, Nino, and his beloved collie, Archibald—and flew to Moscow. "I never thought I would stay in America," he says. "I grew up in Georgia. My home was there. My father was there. My fiancée was there. My family and friends were there. Immigrating to another country? Leaving all of this behind? No, it just wasn't possible."[28]

On October 2, 1993, Sandro boarded a plane from Moscow's Sheremetyevo International Airport to New York. In his luggage, he carried enough clothes to get through the northeastern winter and $500 in cash, all his possessions at that time. A bunch of local yersinia samples for his research were already en route to Baltimore, painstakingly sealed, wrapped, and packaged inside metal containers. He lay back in his seat watching the familiar landscape fly by the window as the plane picked up speed and took off. Little did he know that he was leaving Moscow on the day of a massive constitutional crisis that was already unfurling as he became airborne.

Beginning the month before as a political standoff between the Russian Parliament and President Boris Yeltsin, the dispute escalated, with protestors storming government buildings and the military stepping in. The wheels of Sandro's plane left the tarmac just as Russian tanks rolled onto the Moscow streets. The armed conflict lasted ten days, bringing Russia to the brink of a civil war. While it eventually resolved, the former Soviet empire continued to decline. Sandro had left for good. He just didn't know it yet.

THE PHAGE PHENOMENON

When Sandro climbed out of the puddle jumper that carried him from New York to Baltimore, the entire Morris family, including three young kids, picked him up, treated him to dinner at Baltimore's Inner Harbor, and took him to their house. As they conversed, Morris was impressed by his postdoc's English. "You must've taken a lot of classes with good teachers because you speak really well," he complimented his new fellow.

Sandro shook his head. "I learned English by watching movies," he said.

The next day, Morris's wife, Deborah, helped Sandro settle. With no credit card, no bank account, and no financial history, he couldn't rent an apartment by himself. He couldn't afford one either—the fellowship paid too little. But he earned enough to rent a room in the house of an elderly woman the Morrises knew, which became Sandro's first American home.

Over the next few months, Morris taught Sandro the American ways of life. How to get a driver's license. How to open a bank account. How to write a check. "I didn't know how to take money out of the ATM," Sandro recalls. "Punching the keys on the ATM machine and seeing the green bills slide out was science to me—or more like a miracle, really. I didn't even know how to put gas in the car—not that I had a car when I first got here, but the point is I really couldn't navigate my American life without Glenn."[29]

With bare necessities taken care of, Sandro threw himself into research. Now he had plenty of everything, from equipment to reagents. He worked obsessively, as if trying to compensate for months of forced idleness in his home country. Sandro's *Yersinia bercovieri* species were brewing in the petri dishes of the University of Maryland Infectious Diseases Lab. The bugs were healthy, but the mice infected with them were not. In fact, they got very sick, very fast. Some were already dead, their bellies swollen like birthday balloons. This development was surprising and concerning. *Y. bercovieri* was a close relative to *Y. enterocolitica*, a mild pathogen that causes intestinal distress, but certainly not death. What made *Y. bercovieri* so vicious? Sandro and Morris hypothesized it harbored a novel toxin that its cousin lacked.[30] That meant that *Y. bercovieri* was to be taken much more seriously by the medical community than its less toxic brethren. Sandro and Morris began writing a paper about this phenomenon.

Sandro's discoveries about the peculiar differences between various yersinias' modus operandi were so intriguing that Morris was able to extend his fellowship for a few extra months. When the next term ran out, he did it again. And again. "He was producing some very interesting results," Morris recalls. "So we wanted to continue."[31]

As a microbiologist, Sandro spent most of his time in the lab. Morris, on the contrary, was a physician who tended to patients at the University of Maryland Medical Center. One of the leading infectious disease experts there, he often treated the desperately ill—those who took immunosuppressants after an organ transplant or received chemotherapy that weakened their immune systems, letting infections take hold. Antibiotics were Morris's go-to drugs, but they were starting to fail more and more often. The infections that once were cleared with common medications wouldn't respond even to the more potent ones.

One of Morris's patients, a young man treated for cancer, had been battling an enterococcus infection. An intestinal bacterium that can live peacefully in the human gut, enterococcus has an uncanny ability to cause infections in immune-compromised patients. In hospital settings, it can become resistant to antibiotics, including vancomycin—the drug used to treat it when all else fails. In the mid-1990s, Morris had seen several VRE cases. The young cancer patient was one of them. Despite everything Morris tried, he couldn't save the man.

That afternoon, when Morris dropped into the lab to check in with his research crew, he didn't look like himself. A soft-spoken, kindhearted, confident, and positive person, he was a shadow of his usual self. He seemed strangely aloof. His mind was elsewhere. Sandro asked him what was wrong.

"We lost a patient to VRE," Morris told him with a heavy heart. "After rounds of chemotherapy that wiped out his cancer, he just couldn't fight off enterococcus from his own gut." Like any physician who lost a patient he hoped he could save, Morris felt helpless and useless. "I don't know how to handle these cases," Morris lamented to Sandro. "They don't respond to antibiotics."[32]

Without thinking, Sandro asked a question. "Did a bacteriophage fail too?"

Morris blinked and gave him a blank look. "What bacteriophage?" he asked, dumbfounded. "What are you talking about?"

The other people in the room looked equally perplexed.

It was Sandro's turn to feel perplexed. Clearly, his colleagues would have known about the viral cures for bacterial infections. If his former coworkers still concocted phage cocktails in the war-ravaged, poverty-stricken Tbilisi, successfully treating infections when antibiotics weren't available, the American doctors would have certainly excelled at that.

"I mean, if you can't treat something with antibiotics because of the resistance, you can try a phage, because they kill bacteria with a different mechanism," he went on to elaborate. But Morris was still looking at him with the same what-are-you-talking-about stare. He had no clue what his Georgian fellow meant. "I'd never heard about phage therapy until that conversation," Morris recalls. He had never treated anyone with a phage, nor had any other American doctor he knew.

Sandro was shocked. "It was one of those moments you never forget," he says. "It left a deep impression on me. Somebody just died in the most developed country in the world, after a most sophisticated medical procedure, only because his infection couldn't be treated? Somebody who is a father, a husband, a friend, just died from an infection that could be cured in a developing country like Georgia. It just didn't make sense."

But to American physicians of the early 1990s, the concept of using viruses as medicinal agents didn't make sense. American physicians didn't think of phages as their allies in antibacterial warfare. Morris had known about bacteriophages in nature, but not about their use as living medicines. "How do you know about this?" he asked Sandro.

"The Eliava Institute in Tbilisi has been using phage therapy for decades," Sandro replied. "But the very first time phages were used as medicine was in 1917, in France."

It was Morris's turn to be surprised. He had never heard any of this before.

Sandro realized he had a really big gap to fill, a historical void of about seventy years that spanned from Tbilisi to Paris to Moscow, across the entire Soviet Union, and now all the way to Maryland. "It's a long and complicated story," he said. "But I can tell you everything I know."

2

The Parasite of Microbes

Giorgi Eliava placed a glass slide under his microscope and slowly turned the knob, focusing on the water samples he had brought from the Mtkvari River that flowed through Tiflis—Tbilisi's old name, still used in 1917. Working at the Tiflis Central Laboratory, Eliava was scrutinizing the city's drinking water for the presence of disease-causing organisms. And sure enough, there they were. Under the magnifying lens, the slim, curved rods of *Vibrio cholerae* swam around like self-propelled sausages driven by their wiggly tails. They looked delicate and tender, but they were deadly. The grayish, comma-shaped vibrions turned people into emaciated blue corpses, literally sucking their life out of them.

Sometimes called *blue death*, cholera spread through drinking water, which, without proper treatment, got contaminated by the sewage runoff from leaky pipes, waste gutters, or overflowed outhouses. Once the vibrions settled and multiplied in the human gut, they released a toxin that made the intestinal walls contract violently, expelling water and causing diarrhea, vomiting, and dehydration. The victim's blood pressure and pulse would drop. Their blood would thicken in their veins, starving their body of oxygen—and they would start turning blue. Sometimes they would be dead within hours.[1]

There was no cure, but scientists at the Pasteur Institute in Paris had discovered a way to make cholera vaccines from the dead *V.*

cholerae, so if the bugs were present in the river in large numbers, Tiflis health authorities would be able to start making vaccines. Established in 1888,[2] the Tiflis Pasteur Station had been making rabies vaccines for years, but now the region had to deal with many more plagues.

In the nineteenth and early twentieth centuries, recurring epidemics of cholera claimed hundreds of thousands of lives in Europe, the Middle East, and the Americas, depopulating cities and wiping out entire villages, especially where sanitation was poor. Yet it wasn't the only plague of the time. Dysentery was equally horrifying. Typhus, another lethal bacteria carried by infected fleas, also thrived in the unsanitary conditions. At the time, scientists didn't yet know much about viruses—they were too small to be seen through rudimentary microscopes—but bacterial scourges were deadly. Antibiotics were not yet discovered, so doctors could do little to help patients racked with chills, fever, and diarrhea. Vaccines took time to make and weren't always available.

During World War I, infectious disease outbreaks decimated entire battalions, killing more soldiers than enemy fire. That was the situation Eliava found himself in when, shortly after graduating from Moscow University in 1916, he was sent to the Caucasian war front where the Russian Imperial forces were fighting the Ottomans. The Russian army took over Trebizond, a city in eastern Turkey, but this military success was accompanied by bouts of cholera, dysentery, and typhus. As the lead of the military bacteriological lab that traveled along the front lines, Eliava's duty was to control the outbreaks by vaccinating the soldiers.[3]

A year later, having inoculated enough troops to ensure they wouldn't lose the war, Eliava returned home to Georgia, bringing the laboratory back with him. There he was now, staring at the *V. cholerae* that he fished out from the Mtkvari River. Eliava was not shocked to see them, but not happy either. A few cholera vibrions may not have been a great threat, but when summer arrived and temperatures spiked, the bugs would rapidly proliferate in warm water. If an outbreak happened, did the city have enough resources to mass-produce vaccines to prevent an epidemic?

A knock on the door interrupted Eliava's thoughts. He was being called to yet another meeting. As the laboratory head, he had to participate in many of them. Eliava left the vibrions underneath the lens, locked the lab, and headed out. He had every intention of returning to his work, but the meeting took a while, so he never went back that day. It wasn't unusual for him—he was always torn by an overabundance of ideas and plans, often losing track of time in the process. He was, after all, only twenty-six, and he loved life, every minute of it.

With high cheekbones, light brown hair, an enigmatic smile, and eyes of "the honey hue" that glowed with intellect, Eliava could be irresistibly attractive. Children adored him, women fell in love with him, and men became his best friends. People remembered him as an incredibly eloquent speaker—even when he engaged in a scientific polemic, it sounded like poetry. Unlike most Georgians, he couldn't drink wine—he was allergic—but he had many other ways of enjoying life in his town. A metropolitan city that made Moscow look provincial,[4] Tiflis rivaled European capitals, its architectural beauty lauded by many poets, Georgian and Russian alike. In the 1800s, Mikhail Vorontsov, the czar's deputy to Tiflis, known for his love of arts and culture, built the city by European standards.[5] Tiflis's winding cobblestone streets, charming courtyards, and glass-enclosed terraces earned it the nickname of "Paris of the East," attracting European artists and performers.

Gregarious and full of burning energy, Eliava embraced his city to the fullest. He instinctively knew how to dress, how to court, and how to charm. He appreciated art and literature. He was a passionate dancer and an enthusiastic boxer. He cherished good food and had a sweet tooth—desserts were his favorite part of any meal. He rode horses as if he were born in the saddle, flying across Georgia's beautiful, rugged terrain with snowcapped mountains in the distance. A prankster always ready to pull a joke on a friend, he was forgiven for his disarming ways of doing so. To top it off, he played piano and loved music, so he frequented the opera, where a new star, Amelia Wohl-Lewicka, recently arrived from Warsaw, was performing regularly, enchanting the audience with her lyric-dramatic soprano—a type of voice so powerful, rich, and emotive that it carried easily over a full orchestra. Having recently returned from the war mayhem, Eliava instantly joined the ranks of her admirers and didn't miss a single performance.

Whatever occupied Eliava that evening kept him busy, so he never returned to his lab that night, where his comma-like germs were squirming in the transparent, slowly evaporating water droplets. And in some uncanny way, the bugs were disappearing too, just not quite the same as the H_2O molecules. Little did Eliava know that these vicious microscopic creatures were about to launch his scientific career and his legacy in the world.

I CAN'T BE A DOCTOR!
I CAN'T TAKE MONEY FROM THE SICK

Nicknamed "Gogi," Eliava was born in a small village of Sachkere to the family of a prominent Georgian doctor and grew up in Batumi, a big port city on the Black Sea. Raised in a loving family where his mother and his aunt catered to his every whim, Gogi grew up fearless, accustomed to getting his way. He pursued his interests with ardent passion and was never afraid of the outcome.

He learned to read very early, somewhere between the ages of three and four,[6] and spent hours absorbed in his books. He excelled at playing piano, despite refusing to learn the notation—he had perfect pitch and always played by ear. He could repeat a complex piece of music perfectly after listening to his teacher play it just once. He loved horses, and even the fact that he once fell off and broke his leg didn't stop him from enjoying riding. Later, as an adult, he would buy a purebred in Europe for his own stable.

At fifteen, he graduated the gymnasium—an equivalent of a high school—but wasn't sure what he wanted to pursue in life. He was interested in medicine but didn't think he would make it in the field—he couldn't imagine profiting from human suffering. "I can't be a doctor!" he told his father, the physician. "I will die from hunger because I can't take money from the sick."[7] Whether it was because his father counted Leo Tolstoy among his friends[8] or because of his love for books, Eliava initially decided to study literature.

An idealistic young scholar, he enrolled at Odessa University's Faculty of Philology in 1909. But his literary pursuits ended unexpectedly quickly: Eliava joined the student revolutionary movement, demanding an end to the Russian monarchy. The authorities suppressed the protests and arrested the students. Eliava spent three months in Odessa's jail. More bad news awaited him upon his release—not only was he expelled, he was barred from applying to any Russian university. He had been given a "wolf ticket," as they said in Russian slang—a trip to nowhere.

Shortly after, Eliava's mother, only thirty-five at the time, passed away from pneumonia. To help his children cope with the grief, Eliava's father sent his son and two daughters to Switzerland. The family, affluent and well-connected, hoped that a change of scenery would also help their rebellious scion find his calling in life. The idea worked. Irrepressibly curious, Eliava settled in Geneva at Avenue du Mail, 25, and began auditing classes at the city's university, eventually enrolling at the Faculty of Medicine.[9] Geneva University was known for its liberal views and diversity—it enrolled students from many countries and ethnic groups, including even Jews and women, which many other institutions barred. Eliava's trouble with the Russian government was not an issue.

It was there that he first listened to a microbiology lecture by Hector Cristiani[10] and was captivated by the powerful creatures that seemingly populated every square inch of water and land. For him, it was a different way to practice medicine—not profiting from people's misfortunes but understanding what made them ill and how to restore their health. Knowing bacteria's strengths and weaknesses offered an opportunity to do even more good for humanity than protesting against the czar. It could save millions of lives from infectious diseases. Eliava fell in love with microbiology.

After two years of studying medicine in Geneva, Eliava came home for summer vacation in 1914—and couldn't go back. World War I closed the borders between the Caucasus and Europe, putting his academic degree in peril once again. By that time, the Russian authorities were more concerned with their military actions than mutinous youth, so Eliava's well-connected family convinced those in charge to remove him from the blacklist. Besides, with disease outbreaks raging, scientists and doctors were desperately needed. Eliava was allowed to continue his studies at Moscow University's Faculty of Medicine and then served on the Trebizond front lines before finally returning home to Georgia.

Now, he was chasing cholera vibrions in Mtkvari's water. But this time, a surprise awaited. Having left his experiment unmonitored, Eliava returned to his lab a couple of days later. It was typical of him—he was known for being late for parties, dinners, and even trains. He once showed up at the station only to wave goodbye to the chugging locomotive. This time, he was days late to squint into his microscope to check on his squiggly subjects. To his surprise, he saw nothing on his slide, save for some barely noticeable, unidentifiable dry specks. The water droplets had long since evaporated, but the germs should still have been there, even if they were dead. The lab was locked the entire time, so Eliava was certain that no one had touched his slide or cleaned his equipment. "What happened here?" he wondered, staring at his slide in bewilderment. "Where did they go?" *Something* must have destroyed the microbes. "It could not have been just the Mtkvari water itself, could it?" he asked himself, his curiosity surging.

If nothing else, water would promote the germ's growth. *V. cholerae* naturally dwells in aquatic environments, thriving in brackish or saltwater places where the germs hang on to the chitin-containing shells of crabs, shrimps, and other shellfish. But it doesn't mind freshwater either, which is why it takes hold in rivers and drinking wells. Originally confined to the Indian subcontinent, cholera began hitching rides to new waterways on boats and other vessels after 1817.[11] *V. cholerae* was a hardy, resourceful germ that multiplied with lightning speed. It couldn't just vanish into thin air. Something clearly had extinguished the creatures.

The mystery of the disappearing bugs demanded that Eliava repeat the experiment with full scientific vigor. He grabbed a bucket and headed down to the shore.

Outside, the city was bathed in sunshine and abuzz with activity. Clacking their hooves on the cobblestone streets, donkeys carried provisions to market. Horse-drawn carriages took the Tiflis elite to shop and dine. On the city's main drag, the Golovinsky Prospect (today's Shota Rustaveli Avenue, named after a beloved twelfth-century Georgian poet), strolled elegantly clad couples, stopping at hat shops, flower stalls, and the opera house.[12] The air smelled of blooming lilac, roses, chestnut and cherry trees. Hugging the old, cracked archways, purple bundles of wisteria flowers bent under their own weight, radiating sweetness. Mixed in were puffs of smoke from the wood-burning stoves on which Tiflisians cooked their food—*khachapuri*, the traditional cheesy bread; and *khinkali*, large dumplings filled with delicious juice that are slurped up by hand. Occasionally, the breeze brought in a whiff of sulfur from the bathhouses.

Usually, Mtkvari was a gentle, slow-moving river, leisurely meandering through town, but now it was swollen with spring floods, its green currents rushing down fast. Eliava dipped his bucket and walked back, joining a crowd of water haulers pushing their carts up the hill from the river to the houses that didn't yet have indoor plumbing. But even households that had running water didn't necessarily like cooking with it—many housewives still preferred to get it from Mtkvari. They swore that the food came out different—better, richer, more nuanced. For the sake of convenience, some had switched to making regular meals with tap water but would still procure the Mtkvari goodness from haulers for holiday dinners. To Tiflisians, Mtkvari's taste was superior to running water—it was just too good.[13] And in a way, they were prescient in their assessment.

Back at the lab, Eliava added his water samples to a peptone solution—a form of meat bouillon made with digestive enzymes to make it easier for microbes to eat and grow. He placed the culture into an incubating cabinet and let it sit. A few hours later, when the growing microbes formed a film on the soup—vibrions love oxygen, so they proliferate at the surface—he took a culture swab and placed it under the microscope. Underneath the lens were the classic gray *V. cholerae*, swarming around. Eliava let his culture incubate for a little longer. And then for a little longer still. When he looked again twelve hours later, he could find no traces of the cholera vibrions in his peptone solution.[14] The comma-like germs disappeared without a trace—not only dead but gone entirely, as if they had never been there. "What is this invisible force destroying them?" Eliava racked his brain, now obsessed with the mystery.

He tried another tactic. He planted his Mtkvari vibrions onto an agar plate—another growth medium that serves as bacterial food. He could clearly see them in the dish, which he also left to incubate for a while. But the bugs once again disappeared. When he peered into the plate hours later, the only remnants of the once lively vibrions were the weird spots on the agar's surface: the typically shiny medium lost its luster and appeared matte where the microbes had been.[15] No matter what he did, the phenomenon repeated itself. While starting a normal growth, within a few hours, the vibrio culture would disappear, destroyed by an invisible force. Mtkvari water had indeed proved its goodness. It harbored agents powerful enough to kill cholera, but Eliava's microscope was not acute enough to see them. Something smaller than bacteria was destroying the vibrions. How could this incredibly tiny thing destroy creatures larger than itself? Could he have stumbled onto a new paradigm in microbiology? Or was he simply losing his mind?

In fact, Eliava wasn't deranged. A handful of scientists before him had watched the peculiar disappearance of certain bacterial strains but didn't make special note. They simply wrote it off to laboratory error and moved on. But that was going to change. At about the same time that Eliava was puzzling over the *V. cholerae* disappearance, a different scientist far away, across the war's front lines, observed a similar phenomenon with *Shigella dysenteriae*, the dysentery-causing germ. Named Félix d'Hérelle, he was an assistant at the Pasteur Institute in Paris. And he was certain he had an explanation.

DYSENTERY IN PARIS

At forty-two, Félix d'Hérelle had been at the Pasteur Institute since 1911[16]—during the time when dysentery became a major research interest, ever-more pressing when World War I broke out and soldiers began to fall ill. The Pasteur Institute established a hospital for infectious diseases and d'Hérelle had been trying to understand the modus operandi of S. *dysenteriae*, at the time more commonly called the *bacillus of Shiga*, named after Japanese scientist Kiyoshi Shiga, who discovered it.

Unlike Eliava, d'Hérelle held no degree in microbiology. Born in 1873, either in nearby Montreal, Canada, or someplace in France, or possibly even in Belgium (sources disagree), and raised by his mother in Holland and France, d'Hérelle was a free-spirited, self-taught thinker who never bothered to earn a diploma but was eager to make his mark in science. Much older than Eliava, he had many of the same qualities. He developed a passionate interest in microbiology, was inherently curious, and a "restless world traveler" who seemed to study microbes wherever his peregrinations took him.[17] A Canadian citizen, he was not drafted into the French army but instead worked at the institute making medicines—from antiseptics for wounds to vaccines for rabies and anthrax.

Soldiers at the stalemated French-German front likely started battling dysentery even before Trebizond troops began falling ill with cholera. In the summer of 1915, ten French infantrymen and two civilians stationed in Maisons-Laffitte,[18] in the outskirts of Paris, fell gravely ill with a particularly vicious form of dysentery. Ravaged by bouts of bloody diarrhea, their symptoms were so severe that their doctor, concerned that this new blight could devastate the troops, reported the outbreak to the Pasteur Institute. D'Hérelle, who had previous experience in fieldwork and gastrointestinal maladies, was sent to investigate.

One of his patients arrived very sick but proved luckier than most—he began to recover. As the man got better, d'Hérelle noticed that S. *dysenteriae* began to die out in his stool. He seeded the stool samples onto petri dishes, but despite having plenty of food, shigella didn't prosper much. Instead, some parts of the agar presented small empty spots where shigella had been—just like those matte spots Eliava would later notice. D'Hérelle wrote down his observations, calling them *taches vierges*, or "clear patches."

"The first day, Shiga dysentery bacillus was isolated from the bloody stools but there were no clear patches on the agar of broth culture prepared with the faeces [*sic*] filtrate from the sick person. The same experiment conducted on days two and three were also absent of clear patches." However, on the fourth day, the *taches vierges* finally appeared, indicating that bacteria was being destroyed.[19] D'Hérelle hypothesized that since shigella started dying out in his lab dishes, it would also start withering inside the patient, who would then recover.[20]

By the next morning, he was proven right. The culture, which had been turbid, and thus full of bacteria yesterday evening, was now "perfectly clear; all bacteria had vanished," he wrote. "As for the agar spread, it was devoid of all growth . . . in a flash, I had understood: what caused my clear spots was in fact an invisible microbe," he wrote afterward. "If this is true, the same thing has probably occurred during the night in the sick man . . . He should now be cured. In fact, during the night, his general condition had greatly improved and convalescence was beginning."[21] D'Hérelle was alight with excitement. He essentially foretold that his patient would recover just by looking at the broth culture he had left in the incubator for the night.

Similar to Eliava, d'Hérelle couldn't see the "invisible microbe," but he devised a clever trick to establish its mighty presence. For a few decades, scientists had been using a porcelain strainer with holes so small that fluids could pass through, but bacteria couldn't. Called the Pasteur-Chamberland filter, it was used to purify water and other liquids from microbial organisms. D'Hérelle reasoned that if he passed the bouillon from his petri dishes through the filter, it would remove any and all bacteria but let the smaller agents slip through. He ended up with a clear liquid, seemingly devoid of microbial life. But when he mixed the liquid with shigella in a test tube and left it overnight, the dysentery bugs were gone the next day. Something had clearly lysed them—dissolved their cell walls, so they were bacteria no more.

"They dissolved like sugar in water," d'Hérelle wrote, describing his findings as follows: "I have isolated, from stools and, in one case, from the urine of patients recovering from bacillary dysentery, an invisible microbe endowed with antagonistic effects toward the Shiga bacillus."

It wasn't the first time that researchers caught an invisible substance passing through the Chamberland filter. In the 1890s, two scientists independently investigating the causes of the tobacco mosaic disease found that the microbial culprit slipped through the Chamberland pores and went on to destroy more plant leaves, while remaining invisible under the microscope. They concluded that it was a different form of infectious agent, which they called a *virus*,[22] from the Latin word for "venom" or "poison." And because it wiggled through their state-of-the-art filter, they also referred to it as a *filterable virus*. They did not, however, theorize what this substance was—a bacteria, an enzyme, or some other molecule.

In naming the substance an "invisible microbe," d'Hérelle took the molecular biology a step further. He was so certain because it wasn't the first time that he had seen the phenomenon. A year prior, when he was in Yucatán, Mexico,[23] he witnessed a plague that killed locusts. The insects were dying from diarrhea not unlike human dysentery. Understanding what killed the insects could give humans ways to battle locust infestations. D'Hérelle peered into enough locust poop to notice that sometimes the bacterial culprit, *Bacillus thuringiensis*, would spontaneously lyse too, dissolving entirely and leaving the same *taches vierges* on his agar plates. But the disintegration of the dangerous human pathogen was far more exciting and promising.

D'Hérelle noticed that once all the Shiga bacillus were gone, the "invisible microbe" would go away too. "The anti-Shiga microbe disappears very rapidly following the disappearance of the pathogenic bacillus. Despite numerous attempts, I have never found antagonistic microbes either in the stools of dysenteric patients who are still contaminated or in the stools of normal healthy subjects." Right from the beginning, he had no doubt that these "antagonistic microbes" were, in fact, living creatures rather than bacteria-killing antiseptic compounds like alcohol or enzymes. He was certain they were alive because when dropped into a shigella-seeded dish, they acted like growing colonies of organisms—chewing through and leaving empty spots. That, he wrote, "provides visible proof that the antagonistic effect is produced by a live germ."

He also noticed that the invisible germ refused to grow in any other bacterial culture. "In the absence of dysenteric bacilli, the 'anti-'microbe cannot be cultured in any medium." Neither would it destroy dead bugs, only live ones, d'Hérelle noted. "It does not attack heat-killed dysenteric bacilli." Overall, he concluded that the invisible germ was parasitizing on shigella. "I discovered a parasite of microbes!" he wrote.

D'Hérelle's full description was presented in a paper at the Académie des Sciences by the head of the Pasteur Institute, Emile Roux, on September 15, 1917. Titled "On an Invisible Microbe Antagonistic Toward Dysenteric Bacilli," it described an indiscernible "parasite of bacteria" that devoured the dysentery germ.[24] Published in *Comptes rendus de l'Académie des sciences* (*The Proceedings of the French Academy of Sciences*), an old and prestigious scholarly journal, it was also cited in the French medical weekly *La Presse Médicale*.

Naming this mysterious anti-microbe became a family endeavor. D'Hérelle was married to Marie Caire, a daughter of the French consul in Istanbul, whom he had met on a boat sailing from Europe to Turkey in the spring of 1893. A match for his own adventurous spirit, Marie followed her husband on many microbial quests and became his skilled lab assistant.[25] As the couple's two daughters grew older, they also took part in their father's work. It was with his wife that d'Hérelle first discussed the empty spots in the Shiga culture.

"That night by the lamp, as I related to my family that which I had seen the dysentery bacilli, being devoured by a microbe of microbes, my wife asked what are you going to call it?" he wrote in his memoirs two decades later. The couple spent some time deciding on the name for the obscure yet powerful agent that could hold such incredible immunizing potential. "We searched everywhere proposing and rejecting again and again many names; finally by this collaboration it was 'Bacteriophage' which won out, a word formed from bacteria and *phagein* to eat in Greek."[26] That night's family conversation made history—it coined the scientific term still used a century later.

A bacteriophage parasitizing on human pathogens could make a great ally for humans. Excited by this prospect, d'Hérelle tested his idea on laboratory rabbits. When infected with the Shiga bacteria, the creatures died within five days, but those treated with the bacteriophage recovered with no side effects, leading d'Hérelle to describe his findings as a "veritable 'microbe of immunity.'" If it could cure rabbits, could it also cure humans? It was an electrifying question that d'Hérelle intended to test. He also wondered if nature harbored other bacteriophages that could attack other pathogens—and thought he saw some promising signs. "I was able to observe similar results, though less accentuated, in two cases of paratyphoid fever," he wrote, so "it is probable that this phenomenon is not specific to dysentery, but that it is more widespread."

That's exactly what happened to Eliava's cholera vibrions. But Eliava, who was younger and less experienced, didn't dig deep into the implications. Yet.

FROM PARIS OF THE EAST
TO PARIS OF FRANCE

If World War I had not been tearing Europe apart, d'Hérelle's paper might have reached Eliava. As an affiliate of the Pasteur Institute, the Tiflis Pasteur Station would likely have received the printed periodicals and the article. But during those tumultuous times, Eliava had little access to the academic literature.

Eliava spent some time obsessing over the unexplained mystery, but he eventually put the puzzling phenomenon in the back of his mind. As a medic and a head of the Tiflis Central Laboratory, he was busy with public health measures. And as a young man, he found himself preoccupied with something even more unattainable than microbes: a woman.

A medic and microbiologist who had recently returned from the front, Eliava was elevated to the ranks of a hero, so he was welcomed in all the social engagements in Tiflis—and there were many. At one such gathering, at the home of the elite Dekanozov family, Eliava met a stunning lady. With huge hazel eyes and shiny dark hair, modestly tied on the back of her head, she wore a simple dress and little makeup. She didn't speak Georgian but was fluent in Russian, so the two struck up a conversation about music. Only after a little while did Eliava realize that he was talking to Amelia Wohl-Lewicka, Tiflis's most glamorous opera figure, whose performances

he had been regularly attending. And he was smitten! He wanted
to see her again. And preferably, tête-à-tête.

The legendary lyric-dramatic soprano Amelia Wohl-Lewicka
arrived in the Paris of the East in late 1915 and instantly won the
hearts of the city's music lovers. Equally brilliant as Tatyana in *Eu-
gene Onegin*, Marguerite in *Faust*, or Violetta in *La Traviata*, she
counted thirty-five operas in her repertoire. "She was an elegant,
queen-like lady who commanded respect," says her great-grandson
Dimitry Devdariani, a theater performer in London. When she
went outside for walks, accompanied by her two-year-old daughter, Ganna, and the opera's bookkeeper Pelageya, or Pelo, the
crowds of adoring fans flocked behind. After performances, they
showered their star with lavish bouquets. "The flowers flooded our
apartment to the point that there was no more space to put them,"
Ganna recalled. "With mama's permission, our housekeeper took
some home for herself so they wouldn't wilt in vain."[27]

The glamorous prima donna was married to Nikolay Lewicky,
a voice teacher, who, due to some contractual glitches, was temporarily living in Kyiv, where the couple had originally moved when
running away from the World War I front lines. It was in Kyiv that
the Tiflis opera impresario heard Amelia's voice and immediately
offered her a contract. She signed only after making him promise
that her husband could come too, which Lewicky did a year later.
As beautiful as she was talented, Amelia commanded the stage,
but unlike the stereotypical bohemian diva, she always kept a safe
distance from incessant wooers—a star who could only be adored
from afar. Eliava attended every performance she starred in, diligently adding his bouquets to her blooming heaps.

Amelia's first reaction to the young microbiologist was dispas-
sionate, if not cold. She was used to adoring fans professing their
love. She was accustomed to flower heaps. She was, after all, married to a distinguished theater figure. Finally, she was at least six

years older than Eliava, so she couldn't possibly take his boyishness seriously.

But Gogi was always lucky, and he was going to be lucky again. The spark that once ignited Amelia and Nikolay's romance was dying, even if it wasn't obvious from the outside. Eighteen years her senior, Nikolay had once been everything Amelia wanted to be. Family legend stated that Amelia, born to Jewish parents in Poland, started singing before she learned to talk. She grew up so poor that her father couldn't afford to buy her schoolbooks. Amelia borrowed them from other girls, doing her homework right before class. She managed to graduate from the gymnasium at fifteen with high honors—a silver medal, as Amelia's granddaughter Natalia Devdariani-Malieva remembers. After graduating, she took private singing lessons against her mother's wishes—the older woman believed that the bohemian lifestyle of the theater would turn her daughter into a *fille de joie*. After a while, Amelia began to perform at concerts, where she met the tall, blue-eyed, and exquisitely dressed Nikolay, Warsaw's opera director and a noted voice teacher. Eventually, he proposed, offering Amelia not only his heart but also his expertise in all things music and stage to make her a star. She declined at first, because she refused to convert to Catholicism, but she gave in after a couple of years. As Nikolay's protégée, she signed a contract with the Warsaw opera, where her first performance propelled her to stardom.

After a few years, Nikolay no longer looked like the illustrious character Amelia had first perceived him to be. He could be arrogant, especially to the people of poorer classes, where Amelia herself came from. He had narrow interests and was such a strict father that Ganna disliked and feared him. The move to Tiflis didn't help either. As a performance artist, Amelia had outgrown Nikolay. She was the opera's top star while he was giving lessons at the city's music conservatory. He didn't fit in well either, and because of the language barrier, he preferred a limited company of Polish speakers. Amelia, who had a knack for languages and in addition to Polish spoke fluent French, German, Italian, English, and Russian, enjoyed the company of local socialites and didn't want to confine herself to the Polish diaspora. In fact, she preferred Georgians and fell in love with Tiflis and its people—she found them handsome and warm. She marveled at Georgians' classic beauty—big eyes, chiseled noses, high cheekbones. "Look at that face," she whispered to Pelo, twisting her neck as she gazed at passersby on the street. "Look at the one over there. So many gorgeous people here!"[28]

Gogi took every opportunity to interact with the woman who had become his obsession. He was charmingly insistent about their meetings, playing piano and reciting poetry for her. He had that classic Georgian look she adored, and he was the life and soul of every party, speaking eloquently about Amelia's favorite subjects—art, theater, and music. After attending a concert, he played the pieces he had just listened to from sheer memory.[29] But perhaps most importantly, he was a stark contrast to the stern, cold, and rigid Nikolay. Even little Ganna preferred Gogi's company to that of her father, whom she felt was unreasonably harsh with her.

Weeks and months went by—and the couple found themselves in love. They began meeting at Pelo's place, who also doubled as Ganna's babysitter and insisted on being called Grandma. The older woman reveled in their romance and happily served as a cover to keep the evil gossipers from wagging their tongues. "She began to accompany the lovebirds everywhere to keep Amelia's honor," Ganna wrote in her memoir years later. Sometimes all four of them—the "lovebirds," Pelo, and Ganna—would walk down to the opera house together.

Meanwhile, the world around them was changing. In the fall of 1917, the Russian revolutionary forces had stormed the Winter

Palace in St. Petersburg and overthrown the czar. The new Bolshevik government rushed into a peace treaty with the Ottomans and then with Germany. In May 1918, as the Russian Empire crumbled, Georgia gained its independence. But the victory came with new concerns. As its own country, no longer dependent on the imperial big brother, Georgia now had to supply its citizens with health care and medicine.

In the early twentieth century, medicines weren't made by pharmaceutical giants but rather by research institutions and labs, such as the Pasteur Institute, known for its potent vaccines and serums. As the head of the Tiflis Central Laboratory, Eliava had to make sure that his newly formed, independent country could manufacture the medicines it needed. With military actions in Europe coming to an end, traveling was possible once again. The lab's governing body, the League of Cities, wanted Eliava to go to the Pasteur Institute to learn how to set up a mass production of these remedies[30] at home. Eliava was both excited and proud to be the guardian of his country's health. But his travel plans did complicate his love life.

Eliava begged Amelia to divorce her husband and marry him, but she was desperately torn. Too young, too passionate, too full of too many ideas, Eliava didn't seem ready for a lifetime of commitment. And now, he was talking about a six-month-long research trip to Paris. As if their age difference didn't separate them enough, now there would also be a long, impassable distance. Amelia had her doubts.

But Eliava was passionately insistent. "Mirra, promise me you will be divorced when I return," he demanded, calling Amelia by his affectionate nickname. As the day of his departure approached, they reached an agreement. They were going to get married when Eliava returned.[31] Shortly after, assuring Mirra that he was going to write her letters weekly if not daily, Eliava boarded a train to Batumi, where nearly every ship connecting Asia and Europe docked, towering above the water and smearing blue skies with black soot from their smokestacks. Within days, he watched the waves cresting in the Black Sea as his ship left the port heading for Marseille, full speed ahead in more ways than one.

3

A Georgian in Paris

As he disembarked from the train in Paris, Eliava had no idea that he was about to walk into an explosive scientific controversy. The world of bacteriology did not welcome d'Hérelle's findings of invisible microbes warmly. As a person with no formal microbiology degree, the French scientist found himself on the defensive against an entire scientific universe.

As he continued experimenting with his invisible microbe through 1918, d'Hérelle became convinced that bacteriophages were living organisms that devoured the specific bacteria they parasitized on and therefore could be beneficial to people. That statement alone may not have sounded heretical, because another Pasteur scientist, the Russian-Jewish expat Ilya Metchnikoff, had shown that some bacteria, like acidophilus, was in fact good for human health. But d'Hérelle took it a step further. He theorized that bacteriophages acted as curative entities and "agents of natural immunity." That view contradicted the existing medical doctrine of how immunity worked. According to the established dogma, the human body fought pathogens with an army of specialized molecules and cells—antibodies, leukocytes, macrophages, and other defenders of its own making.[1] Bacteriophages, described as living microbes that no one could see, had no place in that immunity model.

More specifically, d'Hérelle's findings challenged the work of the celebrated scientist Jules Bordet, who had devoted his entire career to immunology and would go on to win the Nobel Prize for his contributions.[2] Bordet, who led his own Pasteur Institute affiliate in Brussels, didn't take the challenge lightly. He and his followers united in vicious opposition to d'Hérelle's view. Some of them legitimately couldn't replicate his experiments. Others argued that phages couldn't possibly be living creatures but were instead the products of patients' immune systems akin to antibodies that attack bacteria, or enzymes that break down bacterial cells. D'Hérelle argued that phages didn't have to be isolated from a patient, because they could exist in nature on their own, but without the clear microscope-produced evidence, he couldn't prove it.

There was even a third camp, which insisted that d'Hérelle wasn't the first one to observe the lysing phenomenon and therefore couldn't even claim the credit. And that argument, indeed, proved true.

It turned out that not one but at least four other scientists had observed a similar bacterial vanishing act as early as twenty years prior. The first was British bacteriologist Ernest Hankin, who in 1896 reported a mysterious antibacterial force floating in the Ganges and Yamuna (Jamuna) Rivers in India that dissolved cholera vibrions and easily slipped through the Chamberland filter. "It is seen that the unboiled water of the Ganges kills the cholera germ in less than 3 hours," Hankin wrote in his paper "The Bactericidal Action of the Waters of the Jamuna and Ganges Rivers on Cholera Microbes." He noted, "The same water, when boiled, does not have the same effect." He went on to produce the following public health recommendation: "The results suggest that during Hindu pilgrimages to sacred places on the banks of the Ganges and the Jamuna, it would be better to advise against the use of well water and encourage use of river water. This would no doubt be easy, as the pilgrims regard this water to be sacred as well as a stimulant for digestion."[3]

Two years later, Russian-Ukrainian microbiologist Nikolai Gamaleia stumbled upon a spontaneous lysis of the dreadful plague bacteria. Another Russian scientist, Waldemar Mordecai Haffkine, who studied the plague in India, also noted that the bugs sometimes disappeared from the prepared culture specimens. In fact, this observation was common enough that his laboratory staff coined a special term for this mystery. "The cultures committed suicide," they joked.[4] And finally, in 1915, only two years before d'Hérelle, British microbiologist Frederick W. Twort wrote about a "transmissible lysis" of microbes, meaning that the lysis could spread from one bacterial colony to the next. But unlike d'Hérelle, none of the other scientists developed their findings into any kind of theory, writing off the strange phenomenon as an unexplained natural wonder or a laboratory mishap.

Nonetheless, the Bordet camp seized on d'Hérelle's mistake of not mentioning Twort's very recent paper and developed it into the "Twort-d'Hérelle Controversy,"[5] trying to disprove his theory. Others just disparaged it. When an employee of Parke Laboratory in New York returned from the Pasteur Institute in 1919 and demonstrated how a bacteriophage solution dissolved microbial cultures, she was ridiculed.[6] In this perfect storm of scientific opposition, the self-taught laboratory assistant with no university degree seemed to stand no chance. A prickly character who spoke his mind and didn't sugarcoat his statements, d'Hérelle's personality didn't help his credibility in the always contrarian, battle-ready, prove-you-wrong scientific ecosphere.

Dealing with global scorn was hard, but life brought d'Hérelle an unexpected, if temporary, escape to the French countryside. In the summer of 1919, he found himself in the middle of another perfect storm, albeit a bacterial one, that only made him more confident in his convictions. The storm once again came in the form of deadly diarrhea, which was devastating chickens.

The bucolic farmland of the Champagne province was rocked by a fatal epidemic of fowl typhoid. Caused by salmonella that had not been seen before in France, the disease apparently arrived from the United States and swept through the poultry flocks like wildfire. After d'Hérelle's inquiry into locust and human digestive disorders, diarrhea in birds was the next logical step, so he headed out to the country hoping to find a curative agent for the new scourge. By that point, he was convinced that the bacteria-bacteriophage relationship should play out in chickens the same way it did in humans. The bird that beat the bug would carry the salmonella-killing bacteriophage, so even one feathery survivor would give him the cure for all.[7]

The typhoid was indeed vicious. For the first four days, d'Hérelle didn't find a single convalescing hen—each and every one of them died. Finally, he caught a break. One hen recovered, and in its feces was the long-awaited bacteriophage that actively destroyed salmonella. D'Hérelle isolated the still-invisible bacteriophage from the hen's droppings and could now give it to all the other sick birds.[8]

That's when things grew even more interesting—d'Hérelle discovered that he didn't even have to treat the rest of the coop. In the henhouse where the recovered bird lived, all her brethren spontaneously recovered too, as if saved by a magic wand. The epidemic stopped instantly. The entire flock now had the salmonella bacteriophage in their feces. One reason why it might have worked so fast was that the birds pecked at each other and their droppings, so as soon as the bacteriophages arrived at the microbial battlefield, they populated the birds in no time. But d'Hérelle also found the same bacteriophages in the feces of other animals and generally around the farm—and deduced that its proliferation caused the cure.[9]

His overall conclusion was that while the sick animals spread the disease, the ones that recovered with the bacteriophage's help could spread the cure. So while the disease was contagious, *the recovery was contagious too*—another radical departure from the established immunological views. Rather than waiting for the bacteriophage to disperse naturally, d'Hérelle proposed that it would be far more useful to spread it artificially, essentially giving it to the sick animals like medicine. It would be a potent way not only to cure the ill individuals but *to end the entire epidemic*, whether among birds, animals, or people. He could now try using bacteriophages as human medicine—if he could only convince his esteemed colleagues that his bacteriophages could indeed act as agents of immunity.

He even had a plan for how to prepare bacteriophage medicine in amounts large enough to give to stricken populations. According to d'Hérelle, this would be simple. Once you isolated the phage that worked against the current germs, you would simply feed the phage more germs in a test tube. The phage would then multiply at the expense of the bacteria. Add more bacteria to the mix—and more phages would grow. Rather than *making* medicines, medics could *grow* them. He fully believed that his idea would work—if he could get anyone to take him seriously.

That was the scientific climate Eliava found himself in as he settled into his new life in Paris. Charming, witty, and well educated, he quickly built a circle of friends. One day, he heard his colleagues discussing d'Hérelle's alleged discovery. Their comments were condescending, if not sarcastic, but their description of d'Hérelle's findings sounded oddly familiar. The bacteria that vanished. The unseen killing force. The specimens that were suddenly clear of germs. The bacteria were different—d'Hérelle was experimenting with Shiga and Eliava with cholera—but the fact that the same phenomenon worked on two different germs was even more exciting.[10] "I believe I have observed the same exact thing," Eliava shared.

His colleagues raised their eyebrows. They already had one funny guy running around with his phage theories of invisible creatures—the institute's laughingstock. Except he was now looking for them in chickens out in the French hinterlands, surely flushing his career down the drain. But Eliava was undeterred. He had identified his next pursuit.[11]

Wasting no time, he went to talk to Emile Roux, the institute's director, who had presented d'Hérelle's paper to the Académie des Sciences in 1917. Eliava told him about his own experiences, his own bewilderment. He said he also suspected the agents of destruction to be microorganisms too small to see. He implored Roux to take it seriously. Always an eloquent and articulate speaker, he asked Roux for permission to repeat the experiments.[12] Roux acquiesced, and Eliava immediately set to work. Here at Pasteur's, he had access to the most up-to-date equipment and the materials he could only dream of back home. He dove headlong into his work, eager to prove d'Hérelle's findings. It didn't matter that he wouldn't be able to claim credit for this discovery—what mattered was making it work.[13] D'Hérelle was still peering into chicken droppings in the Champagne countryside when Eliava began planting germs into petri dishes in Paris.

We do not know exactly what experiments Eliava performed, which could have been on Shiga or cholera. It's not clear where he got the water from or whether he used preserved stool cultures instead. Unlike d'Hérelle, Eliava wasn't meticulous at recordkeeping, so the results from his experiments might have existed only in his scribbly, handwritten notes—or not at all. But the experiments worked. The liquids cleared, and the agar plates displayed the characteristic empty matte spots where the bugs had been only hours before. Eliava managed to fully reproduce d'Hérelle's results. "He staged a series of brilliant experiments," Natalia Devdariani-

Malieva says, recalling the family legend. "And he showed that d'Hérelle was right."[14]

Rumors about a peculiar Georgian who not only sided with the phage theory but had produced convincing proof traveled to the countryside quickly. The father of phages stopped fussing with fowl feces and rushed back to Paris.

Running into the institute, d'Hérelle hollered from the downstairs hallway to his newfound follower so loudly that his voice carried throughout the building. "Where is this Georges Eliava?" he shouted, pronouncing Eliava's name with a French accent. "Show him to me!" Eliava, who was working in one of the labs, ran out to meet the Frenchman. The two hugged and kissed in the middle of the institute hallways, Devdariani-Malieva says. "That meeting was the beginning of their friendship. From that moment on, they were like father and son."[15]

Now d'Hérelle had a phage enthusiast in his own research institution who was equally fascinated by the phenomenon and open to enlisting these powerful allies in the human fight against infectious disease. As a newcomer to the scene, Eliava couldn't possibly quell the opposition entirely, but his belief in d'Hérelle's idea laid the foundation for a lifelong collaboration. Older and more experienced, d'Hérelle became a mentor to the young Georgian during his Parisian stay. And, with Eliava as an ally, he soon got another chance to validate the curative nature of his bacteriophage remedies.

A SMALL GLASS OF PHAGE

In late summer of 1919, dysentery struck once again. The disease had a particular predilection for children, so as another outbreak arrived, d'Hérelle approached pediatrician Victor Henri Hutinel at the Hôpital des Enfants-Malades in Paris with an idea for an experimental treatment. Hutinel was interested. "He agreed to let me treat the young patients on the condition that I first demonstrate that ingestion of the cultures of the bacteriophage were harmless," d'Hérelle wrote.[16] He had no problem with that—he had already drunk numerous loads of phages himself. "I ingested increasing quantities of the cultures, aged from six days to a month, from one to thirty cubic centimeters, without detecting the slightest malaise." He even went so far as to recruit his entire family as phage study subjects with similar outcomes. "Three persons in my family next ingested variable quantities several times without showing the least disturbance,"[17] he wrote afterward.

D'Hérelle proposed that he would once again swallow a hundredfold dose of what he would give to children. Several hospital interns offered to join the experiment too, asking for "a small glass" of phage. "This was probably the first formal phase one human volunteer bacteriophage safety trial ever conducted," says Sandro, who referred to the occurrence in his own work, "but that was fairly typical of the time. Scientists tried their medicines on themselves first."[18]

On August 1, the volunteer group assembled for the test and d'Hérelle passed around a large flask of the bacteriophage brew. Hutinel took a swig too. "Opinion was unanimous, the flavor, if not delicious was not too disagreeable," d'Hérelle had remarked.[19] One day later, none of them had any side effects, so the effort progressed to what today would be the phase one clinical trial—dosing a small cohort with the experimental medicine. Hutinel signed off on the first known therapeutic use of bacteriophages in humans.

Just then, the hospital admitted a very sick twelve-year-old boy, who had been withering from the infection and suffering a dozen bloody stools each day. D'Hérelle treated the child with his cocktail on August 2, and the medics waited for it to work its magic.

And work magic it did. The boy's diarrhea stopped within hours, and by the next morning, all his symptoms were gone. The child, who only yesterday didn't stand a chance to live, recovered literally overnight.

More miraculous cures followed shortly after. About a month later, the hospital admitted three very sick children—brothers aged three, seven, and twelve. Dysentery had already killed their sister, so their own prospects looked grim. After drinking the bacteriophage preparation, all three recovered in twenty-four hours.[20]

Eliava joined the dysentery phage experiments too, but on another level. Instead of drinking the brew, d'Hérelle gave him an injection of bacteriophage culture, after giving one to himself too. "G. Eliava has received by subcutaneous injection 5 cc. of a culture of the anti-Shiga bacteriophage aged thirty days," D'Hérelle wrote. "No reaction, local or general, followed."[21]

In early 1920, d'Hérelle took off on another adventure. When Alexandre Yersin, discoverer of the dreaded plague-causing *Yersinia pestis* germ, visited Paris, d'Hérelle spoke to him about working in Indochina, a group of French territories in Southeast Asia, infamous for their infectious disease burden. D'Hérelle described it as "the land of my dreams: one meets cholera, plague and various epizootics such as the terrible barbone," a cattle disease that had recently killed over a million buffalo within a few months. Yersin, who was the Pasteur Institute director in Saigon, felt that the shortage of bacteriologists in this remote part of the world was hindering scientific progress. D'Hérelle jumped on the opportunity and sailed off to his dreamland shortly thereafter.[22]

Indochina offered the chance to experiment with his bacteriophage applications on all of his dream scourges—cholera, barbone, and even the plague. In September 1920, twelve villagers contracted the disease, and all of them died. Knowing that bubonic plague is spread by rats, who carry the germ without dying and thus must have some resistance, d'Hérelle hypothesized that they might also carry a bacteriophage that fights it. The best place to look for it was in feces, of course, so d'Hérelle added rat droppings to his existing collection of excremental resources. Poking through rat feces proved successful—he isolated an extremely potent anti-plague bacteriophage. He was convinced that he now held the cure for the plague—the disease that famously had no cures. All he needed was a chance to use it. And in the near future, he would get that chance.[23]

IN LOVE, DIVIDED

Meanwhile, Eliava was busy in Paris. Among other things, he was working in the laboratory of Edouard Pozerski, a Polish scientist who had become his good friend. Eliava came to the Pasteur Institute to study the production of vaccines and serums, and there was plenty to learn. The six months he had originally promised Amelia flew by, and he wasn't going home yet. Busy and easily distracted with ideas and projects, he wrote more sporadically than Amelia would have liked. Making things worse, letters took weeks or even months to arrive. Even when the Great War finally ended at the close of 1918, the international mail infrastructure was in shambles. Ganna wrote that some letters made it to Tiflis only because some helpful friends at the French consulate passed them along with important mail or with human travelers.

Gogi's unwieldy penmanship was even harder to follow than the multitude of his ideas, so Amelia spent hours trying to piece together the meanings of his long-awaited messages. "I remember my mother crying her heart out over one of these precious letters because she couldn't understand his handwriting," Ganna would later say. And because their relationship still wasn't official, she didn't want to ask anyone for help. Soon, even those infrequent messages from Gogi stopped arriving, and Amelia no longer knew whether he was ever coming back. With a heavy heart, she plowed on. She still performed at the opera and Nikolay still taught music lessons, but their relationship crumbled just like the world around them. Food shortages grew more and more common. The theater struggled with money. Performances foundered because even the most devoted patrons couldn't afford tickets. None of that helped the couple that no longer found comfort in each other's presence. Ganna remembered her parents' dramatic disputes. "After one of their heated conversations, my father left the apartment and sat on the stairs, weeping, so my mother sent me to console him."

The circulating rumors of the Red Army approaching Georgia, as well as the horrifying tales of the terror they would inevitably bring, made things even more depressing. The rumors were far from unfounded—following Vladimir Lenin's idea of the dictatorship of the proletariat, the Bolsheviks stopped at nothing in their path to power and had already earned a reputation as bloody and ruthless terrorists. They confiscated people's possessions, throwing citizens out of their homes and shooting parents in front of children. To assure that civilians, drafted into the Red Army against their will, fought fiercely in combat, the Bolsheviks used the same decimating tactic as the Romans. If a group retreated from the battleground, the commissars lined up the soldiers and shot every tenth one. Even the name *Red Army* drew its origin in the color of blood. The recently independent Georgia was no match for the wrath of the Reds.

As Polish citizens, Amelia and Nikolay could return to Warsaw now that the war had ended. Yet in the battered, utterly disconnected world of the early twentieth century, that meant that Amelia would likely never see Gogi again. But was it even realistic to expect him to return? Young, attractive, and single in Paris—how much of a chance did she stand of him remembering her, after all this time? And why would he consider returning to Georgia when he could stay in France?

In 1920, the struggling couple moved to a new apartment, nearby the conservatory where Nikolay gave lessons. It was an airy three-bedroom on the first floor overlooking the street. "In February 1921, from the balcony of this apartment, I watched the Red cavalry proudly parading in a victorious procession along the Golovinsky Prospect," Ganna recalled. The Paris of the East wasn't going to retain its Parisian flair much longer, and many wondered if they had waited too long to leave.

DESTINED FOR DESTRUCTION

The beginning of 1921 was fateful for Eliava as well, albeit for different reasons. He began working closely with d'Hérelle again, who had finally returned from Southeast Asia. After spending almost a year in the Far East, d'Hérelle came back in great spirits, excited to thoroughly test his new knowledge—only to discover that he no longer had a lab space. Even though his position of laboratory chief had remained intact, his workspace was taken away. "The reception which I had at the Pasteur Institute was very different than what I had the right to expect," he lamented.

In d'Hérelle's absence, the institute's leadership had changed. Roux was replaced by Albert Calmette, who didn't like d'Hérelle. Calmette had been working on a vaccine against tuberculosis for children and was planning to start administering it. The vaccine, named *Bacillus Calmette–Guérin,* used an attenuated but still living germ, *Mycobacterium bovis,*[24] and some scientists, including d'Hérelle, argued that it wasn't safe. "I thought that attenuated but living bacteria which constituted BCG did not maintain their weakened state in the young organisms but recovered little by little the virulence and did not prevent the formations of lesions by the time the child reached the critical age for tuberculosis, adolescence," d'Hérelle wrote. When he returned from Southeast Asia, Calmette asked him whether he considered the BCG dangerous, and d'Hérelle, never smooth when it came to science politics, answered point-blank that he did. D'Hérelle knew Calmette didn't take his "dissent" well. "Beginning at that moment he swore toward me with implacable hatred."[25]

D'Hérelle asked Roux for another laboratory space but got nowhere. "He responded that none were available at that moment and that besides this was now Calmette's responsibility," he later recalled. "In spite of it all, I continued to work. A friend, Pozerski, had given me the use of a corner of a table in his minuscule laboratory."[26] It was the same Edouard Pozerski that had befriended Eliava.

It was in that "minuscule laboratory" that d'Hérelle and Eliava worked together setting up various experiments to study bacteriophages' behavior, accumulating proof that they were living organisms actively attacking other creatures. They couldn't see phages doing their "tailwork," but they saw the results. Under their simple microscopes, they watched the most amazing microbial massacre, at least by the early-twentieth-century standards, which d'Hérelle would later describe in detail in his book *The Bacteriophage: Its Role in Immunity*.

Infected by a phage, the bacteria, happily floating in a bouillon solution, would start to swell. They would change their normal shapes from rodlike to spherical, slowly turning into fat, round blobs. One could almost feel the immense force pressing on their cell walls from the inside—until the membranes finally gave out and the bacteria exploded, spitting out microscopic debris—and the next generation of invisible invaders.

"If the spherical bodies are observed with care it is seen that after a variable length of time, sometimes amounting to only about ten minutes, an actual bursting takes place, consuming but a fraction of a second," d'Hérelle wrote, summarizing the experiment. "Immediately afterward, in the place of the spherical body there remains a slight cloudy floccule that slowly dissolves, thus liberating the fine granules. These spherical bodies are particularly abundant at the time when the lytic process is at its maximum rate. There can be no question concerning the nature of these bodies; they are bacilli which, operated upon by a force which can only be internal, take at first a globoid form and then rupture." Destruction of the bacilli would look completely different if the dissolving action was done from their exterior, d'Hérelle noted. "The spherical form and the bursting prove beyond possible contradiction that the operating force is internal,"[27] he stressed as a proof that the microbes weren't being chewed up by enzymes or immune system molecules. They blew up because of the internal parasites that invaded and multiplied and then destroyed their hosts.

Cell after cell followed the same path, defenseless against the phages. Peering into the microscopes, the scientists could see the microbes' defeat and the sad remains of their bodies floating, suspended in the liquid. The one and only thing they couldn't see was their slayer, the "ultramicrobe."[28] Not until the 1930s would scientists be able to see viruses using electronic microscopes, but the phage enthusiasts were prescient enough to theorize that their study subjects latched on to the bacterial cells, squeezed themselves inside, and multiplied within until they were ready to break through. "The culture of the ultramicrobes takes place within the interior of the bacillary body . . . Each of the ultramicrobes inoculated penetrates to the interior of a bacillus and there multiplies up to the time when the bacillary body bursts. This liberates the colony of ultramicrobes which have been formed in the bacterial protoplasm."[29]

Some bacterial cells that held on to their defenses longer would eventually meet their end. It was a matter of time, of the initial ratios of bugs and bacteriophages and sometimes of temperature—but there was no escaping that ultimate, unforgiving destruction. Once "inoculated" with phages, the microbial community was destined for death. "It has been seen that when the inoculation with the bacteriophage is massive all the bacteria are attacked at the beginning, in other words, their multiplication is abruptly arrested. After two to three hours, the medium commences to clear little by little and becomes completely limpid a short time later. If, on the contrary, the inoculation is minimal, the few ultramicrobes inoculated only affect an equal number of bacteria. The great majority remain unaffected and multiply as they would in a normal medium. But the ultramicrobes likewise multiply, following a progression more rapid than that pursued by the bacteria, so that within a few hours their number becomes equal to, or greater than, that of the bacteria. This is the time when macroscopic lysis commences."[30] After several hours, the microscopic rubble would disappear, leaving behind a clear liquid as if the germs were never there. "After thirty-six hours nothing whatever can be distinguished."[31]

In his book, d'Hérelle deliberated about where in the animal kingdom the bacteriophage belonged. "Is it a protozoan? Is it a bacterium? Does it belong to a kingdom which is neither vegetable nor animal?" he questioned. Once again, he was prescient—because many modern scientists still subscribe to the idea that viruses are neither dead nor alive. "It is an ultramicrobe, a filtrable being endowed with the functions of assimilation and of reproduction, functions which characterize the living nature of beings and which pertain to them alone." Based on where he first found it, d'Hérelle gave his discovery a full Latin name, *Bacteriophagum intestinale*.[32]

In April 1921, just as the Bolsheviks' cavalry was parading outside Amelia's windows, filling Tiflisians with dread, d'Hérelle and Eliava published a joint paper in which they argued with Bordet's camp that phages were living entities. The proof was a convoluted set of experiments aimed to show that even though the phages' ability to dissolve bacterial cells could be temporarily inhibited by some chemicals, eventually, they would resume their feast. To the two phage enthusiasts, it was a clear sign that phages weren't enzymes or immune system molecules, because only living beings could restore their appetite and their "consuming properties."

D'Hérelle's other argument that phages weren't produced by the immune system was that they existed in nature on their own. His work in Southeast Asia convinced him that bacteriophages not only dwell everywhere on earth but that every germ on the planet likely has its own bacteriophage enemy—and that phages would make great allies for humans.

He was prescient once again. Today, we know that bacteriophages are some of the most abundant entities on earth. They are found wherever bacteria dwell, meaning everywhere, in the atmosphere, in the soil, and in the water. Ernest Hankin, who recommended drinking water from the Yamuna and Ganges rather than from the wells, was correct—the rivers were indeed teeming with phages that kept them potable. While villages routinely floated their dead in the rivers' holy water, the cholera outbreaks along the shores were rare and few, and significantly less deadly than those in the West. The phages devoured the vibrions, preventing them from traveling downstream. That purifying quality had likely led to the Yamuna's and Ganges's holy status. Because of the rivers' unique biology, Hindus, who washed in their waters along with their farm animals, and drank that same water afterward, were indeed better protected from the disease.

Another place rich with phages is sewage—because it's teeming with an abundance of bacteria that provide plenty of food for a variety of their eaters. Animals and humans are full of bacteriophages as well—they are part of our normal virome, a viral equivalent to the microbiome. Phages dwell on us and inside us, on our skin, in our mucus and our guts. They live in the intestines of all living things that have a digestive tract and can be found in the stools of healthy individuals. Moreover, we owe that good state of health to them, at least in part. By populating us, they indeed act as "agents of natural immunity," as d'Hérelle described them, defending us from the pathogenic bugs that cross our paths. When phages wither, so do we, because we lose that protection—the natural immunity they bring. And as the two pioneering scientists presciently concluded, administering phages can restore or bolster that immunity.

Working together, they began to lay the foundation for manufacturing phage-based medicines. To administer phages as therapeutic agents, they needed to establish proper doses and schedules. They also had to establish the limits of phage power. What would kill a particular phage? What would diminish its lysing potency? How long would phages live in a solution devoid of their bacterial food before becoming ineffective? Can a dysentery or cholera phage evolve or be "trained" to attack other bacteria if it spends enough time "in their company"? Toiling in the little space they had, d'Hérelle and Eliava, sometimes with their friend and lab chief Pozerski, searched for answers.

Alcohol, they found, killed bacteriophages. And, unlike bacteria, bacteriophages were very sensitive to quinine, commonly used against the malaria parasite. "Eliava and Pozerski have shown that the neutral salts of quinine exert an antiseptic action on the bacteriophage, in three per cent solution killing it in thirty minutes, in one per cent, in a few hours," d'Hérelle acknowledged. That was an important find, helpful with isolating a pure bacterial culture untainted by any bacteriophages for future experiments. D'Hérelle included the instructions in his book. "An ultrapure bacterial culture can also be obtained by the use of quinine, since this substance has a higher antiseptic activity for the bacteriophage than for the bacterium."

D'Hérelle credited Eliava with a number of experiments—if this was a modern paper he would have been listed as a collaborator. Working with a bacteriophage isolated from the pus of an abscess, Eliava found it to be very potent against *Staphylococcus aureus*—a bacteria still dreaded to this day. *S. aureus* can dwell on human skin until it suddenly becomes destructive, causing boils and other infections, and can be deadly if it gets into the bloodstream. Its methicillin-resistant *Staphylococcus aureus* strain, the notorious MRSA, still kills about twenty thousand Americans each year.[33] Yet in the early 1920s, Eliava was experimenting with a phage capable of destroying it. Moreover, according to d'Hérelle's notes, he was trying—with some success—to train that phage to develop "a degree of activity for the dysentery bacillus."[34]

Impressed with Eliava's scientific acumen and intuition, so similar to his own, d'Hérelle suggested he should stay at the Pasteur facility. With his talents—and a prestigious bacteriology degree to his name—Eliava was certain to do quite well. He had already published papers. His name was going to appear in *The Bacteriophage: Its Role in Immunity*, which d'Hérelle managed to get to print—Roux pushed it through while Calmette was on vacation. Published in 1921, it was translated in English by George H. Smith, assistant professor of bacteriology at Yale School of Medicine, and would be widely read by English-speaking bacteriologists. If Eliava wanted to stay in Paris, he certainly could. There were ways to make it happen.

By early 1921, when the Bolshevik cavalry stormed into Tiflis, Eliava had been gone for over two years, and Amelia had finally lost faith that he would ever return.

ALL ROADS LEAD TO BATUMI

At first, at least, the new Bolshevik government proved fairly benevolent, allowing the Polish diaspora to return to their homeland. It took multiple trains to transport the Polish community to Batumi, where they would board a ship to Europe.

Only at the end of the summer, with the very last train scheduled to depart Tiflis, did Amelia finally decide to leave. She gave her farewell performance at the opera, lit by a flickering kerosene lamp standing on the piano because the electricity no longer worked. The audience wouldn't let Wohl-Lewicka off the stage, begging her for endless encores. "Someone delivered a passionate speech, asking mama not to leave Tiflis," Ganna recalled. "By the end, the speaker, the singer, and the audience were in tears. They sobbed so hard you could hear them down the hall."[35]

Amelia left with a heavy heart. She didn't want to go to Warsaw. She didn't want to start her life and career anew again. She had already done it twice, running away from the war and falling in love with Gogi. Now her love abandoned her, her family fell apart, and her theater career was in shambles once more. Nikolay wasn't coming home with her. By then, he had a mistress, one of his students at the conservatory.

The last Batumi-bound train was a freight with no berths, no rooms, and no restrooms. Amelia and Ganna slept on two trunks packed with their belongings, piling clothes and linens to cushion their makeshift beds. Many of Amelia's admirers were on the same abysmal journey.

Today, the ride from Tbilisi to Batumi takes five hours, but in 1921, it took eight days, because the train often stopped and waited for locomotives to pass. In Batumi, the migrants expected to transfer to a steamboat named *Albania*, the only one that agreed to transport them back home. The steamboat hadn't arrived yet, so the travelers had to find temporary places to stay. They rented rooms and waited. Days came and went, but the ship wasn't anywhere in sight, so the displaced community developed a routine. Every morning, they walked along the shore, gazing into the horizon where the sky kissed the sea, in search of the long-awaited vessel, trying to discern the outline of a smokestack, dark puffs of fumes, anything. Two weeks passed.[36]

It was on a perfectly beautiful morning that Amelia and Ganna heard news of an arriving ship. Together with Amelia's friend, they rushed to the port, only to learn that it wasn't the long-awaited *Albania* but a different ship arriving from Marseille. Holding on to her mother's hand, wide-eyed Ganna looked up at the deck crowded by the passengers waiting to get off. Among them, she spotted a familiar figure.

"Mama, Mama, look!" she shouted, pointing up in excitement. On the deck stood the man who used to play with her and bring her treats. "It's Dr. Eliava!"

Amelia gasped. To her, the ship's deck was all but a blur—she was too nearsighted to see anything at a distance. "For the love of god, please tell me it's him," she cried out to her friend.

The woman looked up. There, beyond any doubt, stood Eliava, fervently waving his hat at the female trio down below. "It's he," the woman friend confirmed. "It's Gogi!"[37]

Amelia didn't know what to do. In her mind, she all but had let Gogi go. And what if he was no longer interested in her? She was too nervous to face him in public, waiting among the crowd as the passengers shuffled through customs. "Please tell him where to find me, but only if he asks!" Amelia told her friend and headed home with Ganna. There, she sat and waited, anxiety thrumming in her chest. What would she do if he didn't come? What would she say if he did?[38]

She waited for a long time. It was so long that she decided Gogi wasn't going to come at all. And he, in fact, had gone to see another woman first—his younger sister, who lived in Batumi and who had been sick for a long time. Having learned that she passed away, Gogi rushed to the cemetery with a heap of flowers—and then to find the love of his life.

Their first meeting in two years was tender and dramatic. Gogi begged Amelia not to go home and to marry him instead. He was devastated that she was still married to Nikolay and feverishly upset that she had waited so long.

"You promised me that you would be divorced when I returned," he fumed, heartbroken and jealous. "Why are you still with this man? Do you still love him?"

"You were gone for two years," Amelia retorted. "I didn't know if you were ever going to come back."

"How could you not trust me? Or you don't love me as much as you loved him?" Gogi had always planned to come back. This was his home, his family, his Georgia. He left to learn how to help his country and its people to stay healthy and fight disease. "Of course I would return!"[39]

After several days of tears and conversations, Gogi convinced Amelia to stay. He left for Tiflis to find a new apartment big enough to fit his family while she and Ganna remained in their rented Batumi place. Shortly after, Nikolay came to see his daughter—and tried to persuade her to come to Warsaw with him. "I remember us walking along a deserted seashore on a dreary rainy day, enveloped in fog swirling from the water. He talked about how much he loved me and how much he was going to miss me. He promised me toys, sweets, and my own room. But all I did was keep looking around for people, horrified that he actually might take me away with him—and I will never see my beloved mother again. Thankfully, he left and I stayed."[40]

It took Eliava several months to set up a home for his new family. He had too many things demanding his attention. He had to organize the production of Georgia's own medicines—a gargantuan task in the postwar era. It wasn't until May 1922 that Gogi and Mirra reunited once again. It was a lovely season to rekindle the romance. Tiflis was in full bloom, and florists sold bouquets on every corner.

A month prior, Joseph Stalin had succeeded Vladimir Lenin as the leader of the new Soviet state. A Georgian himself, with the real last name Jughashvili, he was partial to his old homeland. At least for now, he was ready to support science and see Georgia prosper under his rule.

4

Phages Rise to Fame and Glory

The apartment Gogi found for his new family overlooked a charming street lined by beautiful old mansions. It occupied two floors, had three spacious bedrooms, a guest room, and a classic Tiflis courtyard surrounded by greenery, where the family dined in summers. The master bedroom was hand-painted with a mural of a blooming garden depicting trees rising to the ceiling and flowers climbing the doors. The apartment was mostly furnished, but Gogi immediately bought two essential pieces—a new bed and a grand piano.

Amelia's divorce unfurled into a bitter custody battle. Although Ganna never felt her father loved her, he fought viciously to take her to Poland by portraying Amelia as an unfit mother because she left him for another man. Ganna was dragged into the maelstrom—Tiflis's judicial authorities questioned her about her parents. With no desire to live in Warsaw with her father, she insisted on staying with her new family. The battle raged on until Amelia's lawyer—Eliava's relative—finally won the fight with an irrefutable argument: "It would do a young child a great disservice to miss out on the experience of the great Socialist Society." With that, Nikolay had lost the case and left for Poland with his new wife.

Gogi married Amelia and adopted Ganna, who assumed both his last name and his *otchestvo*, his middle name. In Russian tradition, middle names are not given but inherited from one's father for male and female children alike, with only a slight difference in the ending indicative of gender. As Ganna Giorgievna Eliava, she considered Gogi her only father and remembered him as a caring and loving person. As a husband, however, Gogi was more difficult. He was extremely jealous and for a while couldn't forgive Amelia for not divorcing Nikolay while he was away. It pained him so much that at some point, Amelia, concerned that he might harm himself, hid his revolver inside a fireplace of Ganna's bedroom. When an opera impresario invited Amelia for the next show season, Gogi insisted that she perform as Eliava and not Wohl-Lewicka. The shocked impresario argued that the public wanted to hear their star Wohl-Lewicka, but Amelia, yielding to Gogi's demands, refused. The contract fell apart, and she essentially left the theater, performing only in occasional concerts and in the company of friends—a move she bitterly regretted later, says Natalia Devdariani-Malieva. "She was too much in love with Gogi at that time."[1]

As the head of the Tiflis Central Laboratory, Eliava was brilliant and enthusiastic. For all their brutal acts in taking power, the Bolsheviks considered medical services not a business but a basic human right, so all tests and treatments were provided free. In the new socialist reality, Eliava's childhood worry about profiting from the sick didn't apply—the government paid for everything, so he could do his work without guilt, and he threw himself into it.

From the Pasteur Institute, Eliava brought a shipment of serums, vaccines, reagents, and laboratory equipment worth 100,000 francs. That was a start, but the much-needed remedies weren't going to last forever. The Tiflis Central Laboratory had to meet the growing demand for medicines, and by 1921, it was already responsible for making a certain amount of smallpox and cholera vaccines not only for Georgia but for other Caucasus regions and the Red Army troops. Following an outbreak of typhoid fever, the lab began producing typhoid vaccines, packaging them in ampoules and shipping them by the thousands. But the real challenge was making vaccines in the required amounts when an outbreak hit.

Quickly ramping up production required a readily available supply of raw reagents and people who understood chemistry and biology. Reagents were hard to procure, and qualified personnel were in even shorter supply—in the postrevolutionary chaos, there just weren't enough college graduates looking for jobs. However, because the Soviets embraced gender equality, the myth that girls didn't belong in science was dispelled, so many of Eliava's hires were women. His gender-agnostic employment practices laid the foundation for the organization's future. In the years that followed, female employees, students, and doctoral candidates commonly outnumbered male ones, notes Nina Chanishvili, the head of the Laboratory of Microbial Biotechnology at the Eliava Institute and its de facto historian.

Despite its challenges, the Tiflis Central Laboratory did well, earning a nod of approval from the People's Commissariat of Health. (The fledgling USSR, with Georgia as its republic, was now governed by a series of Narodniy Komitets, or People's Commissariats, with the name stemming from the fact that all decisions—financial, health, or education—were made by the people and for the people.) "Ten months after the launch date, the Tiflis Central Laboratory proved its practical and scientific importance. Led by Dr. Eliava, the laboratory personnel managed to achieve the necessary goals, despite shortage of equipment and other issues,"[2] read the commissariat's report.

To meet Georgia's health care demands, Eliava proposed to expand the lab into the Bacteriological Institute. He had ambitious goals for his brainchild—from upping vaccine and serum production to studying Georgia's native microorganisms, pathogenic and not. The institute would also diagnose and treat patients. In Eliava's vision, it was to become a clinic, a pharmaceutical plant, and a research institution, all in one. Abbreviated as NarKomZdrav, the People's Commissariat of Health approved the creation of the Bacteriological Institute and Eliava's financial estimates on November 10, 1922. It even set the opening date—Saturday, November 18, 1922, only eight days ahead. In reality, the institute opened a few months later, on February 21, 1923. Its structure and departments—research, diagnostic, treatment, prophylactic, and manufacturing, some of which were led by doctors Eliava worked with on the Trebizond front lines—reflected his vision. The institute advertised its services to the people and kept records of how many it served.[3] A year later, it produced enough medicines to sustain the Georgian Republic, earning another NarKomZdrav nod. "The Bacteriological Institute played an important role in fighting infectious disease, having increased the production of vaccines and serums to the point that it is no longer necessary to import them from abroad; almost everything is now made domestically."[4]

In March of 1924, the People's Commissariat decided to house the institute in a centrally located three-storied building on 4 Machabeli Street. But the institute needed more room—and not just office or bench space. It needed a place for stables and barns.

At the time, many medicines were produced using animals that weren't susceptible to the infections that ravaged people. For vaccines, scientists used either dead bacteria or bacterial toxins to elicit an antibody response, preparing people's immune systems for real pathogens. But the so-called serums—the medicinal cocktails that neutralized bacteria or their toxins—were typically derived from animals invulnerable to the germs. A serum for diphtheria—an often-deadly childhood infection that covered throats in phlegm, depriving victims of oxygen and damaging their hearts with toxins—was made by injecting horses with the bacteria *Corynebacterium diphtheriae*. The horses didn't succumb to the infection but instead produced antitoxins, which medics harvested from their blood, purified, and used to treat wheezing and suffocating children, often bringing them back from the brink of death. A serum for treating tetanus, a common and often lethal illness caused by the bacteria *Clostridium tetani*, the spores of which dwell everywhere from dust to soil to rusty nails, was produced in a similar way.

The laboratory needed to build a facility to house the horses to make diphtheria and tetanus serums, as well as young calves used in the production of smallpox vaccines. To sustain mass production, the facility had to keep a substantial number of animals, which wasn't possible in the city center. Eliava petitioned the authorities for a large piece of land in Saburtalo, then a plot on the city's outskirts and now a part of Tbilisi. Occupied by cherry gardens, it stretched along the shores of the Mtkvari, which harbored phages in its currents, offering another convenience. The NarKomFin—People's Commissariat of Finances—acquiesced, giving Eliava 25,000 rubles to start construction.[5] The first buildings erected in Saburtalo were the horse stables.

In the postrevolutionary, war-ravaged reality, money and resources for Eliava's plans were tight. To forge ahead, he had to wage many battles with the NarKomFin, justifying every ruble spent. His speaking talents saved the day more than once. Often, he won on sheer passion, charming his opponents into his visions. Once, when a commissariat's representative declined Eliava's estimated budget as ridiculously exorbitant, Eliava launched into such a passionate speech that he irrefutably proved his case, completely disarming his opponent. The man didn't bear any grudge—he just footed the bill, and from that point, they became close friends.[6]

Eliava and his staff also worked on educating the region's doctors on the latest developments in microbiology, covering a range of subjects: "Bacteriophages' Existence in Tiflis," "The

Latest Diagnostic Methods for Syphilis," "Review of d'Hérelle's Bacteriophages."

The living medicines were dominant in Eliava's mind. But consumed with the institute's daily grind, he didn't have enough time to do research. There was, however, the need to keep up with the quickly developing fields of microbiology, so in 1925, Eliava was dispatched to the Pasteur Institute once again. Unfortunately, by the time he arrived there, his old friend had departed, fighting one of the worst diseases afflicting humans. D'Hérelle finally got the chance to use the plague bacteriophage he had long ago extracted from rat feces—albeit far, far away.

THE RAT FECES CURE

Georges Cap fell ill on July 10, 1925, while on a ship that recently arrived in Alexandria, Egypt. The eighteen-year-old traveler had a bad headache and a surging fever, and was dizzy and exhausted. By the next day, he developed two ominous swellings on his legs. Called *buboes*, a common name for enlarged lymph nodes, they were a characteristic sign of the bubonic plague, also known as the infamous Black Death, which spread via infected fleas and killed nearly everyone who contracted it. The buboes usually developed near the bite sites and, together with fever and fatigue, signaled grim prospects for patients and health authorities because the first case would hardly be the last. Cap was promptly taken off the boat and brought to a nearby hospital tasked with ensuring that diseases arriving on ships didn't spread to town.[7] The worries intensified as three more cases followed shortly after. D'Hérelle, stationed at the port as a guardian of infectious cases, was called to the scene.

Cap deteriorated quickly. By day three, he was unconscious

with a fever of 40.3°C (104.5°F) and heart rate of 130. The young man's survival chances were close to zero, but d'Hérelle believed he could save him. The bacteriophage he had extracted from the rodents' droppings in Southeast Asia still had a strong virulence—the attack-and-destroy power—against the bacteria. On July 13, the young man was sprawled on the hospital bed in such feverish delirium that he didn't even react to the needle as d'Hérelle jabbed the syringe of the bacteriophage solution into his swollen flesh. "I gave an injection of .5 CC of Pestis-bacteriophage into each of the two buboes, the needle being introduced about the center of each bubo," d'Hérelle wrote in his notes, a diligent record-keeper as always. "Apparently the injection caused no pain since the patient showed no reactions of defense."[8] Then he waited for the phages to work their magic again.

And they did, with the same remarkable speed. By the next morning, the patient felt better. He was still weak, but no longer in pain, except when pressing on the still sensitive buboes. "On July 15th, he sat up in bed; and on the 16th he begged for food,"[9] d'Hérelle observed. By then, the second patient had developed high fevers and buboes, so d'Hérelle treated him the same way, with similar results. "Several hours after the injection the patient stated that he felt much better, fell asleep and woke up in the morning with the claim that he had been cured."[10]

Using a syringe, d'Hérelle extracted a few drops of bloody fluids from the patients' buboes, in which he failed to find any bacterial culture. The bacteriophages had devoured absolutely all the *Yersinia* bugs—to the point that when d'Hérelle injected the fluids into a guinea pig, it developed no infection, still alive and well ten days later—a surprising outcome. On the contrary, bacteriophages were plentiful in the sample, having multiplied at the expense of the destroyed germs. D'Hérelle treated the remaining patients with similarly spectacular results, which were reported in the lead article of the French weekly *La Presse Médicale* on October 22, 1925.[11]

News spread quickly about the potent medicine that cured the scourge that had nearly depopulated Europe in the Middle Ages. The British representative of the Conseil Sanitaire, a local health authority, wrote to his superiors that with the arrival of the bacteriophage, the dread of plague may be finally over—and other countries should take note. "Dr. d'Herelle had already supplied Sanitary Administration of Egypt with the necessary bacteriophage. I think India ought to arm itself, also all countries where plague prevails. All honor to d'Herelle. I'm proud of having introduced him to Egypt."[12]

D'Hérelle had arrived in Alexandria in 1924, after spending three fruitful research years in the University of Leiden in the Netherlands. In the fall of 1921, shortly after his book *The Bacteriophage: Its Role in Immunity* was published, a delegation of three professors from Leiden came to Paris and asked d'Hérelle to join their newly formed Institute of Tropical Medicine.[13] The institute's director, Paul Christiaan Flu, originally from Indonesia, wanted to explore the idea of using phages as a prophylactic means of cleaning public water supplies, very often contaminated by bacterial pathogens. Not happy at Pasteur's, d'Hérelle accepted the offer and soon moved his family to Leiden. They settled in Noordwijk, a small village by the North Sea, about the same time that Eliava and Amelia reunited in Tiflis in their new garden-like master bedroom.[14]

Netherlanders appreciated d'Hérelle's vision for medicine far more than any of his previous European colleagues had. Within a few years, he had received several highly coveted tokens of scientific appreciation. With Flu's recommendation, the University of Leiden awarded him an honorary medical degree. The Royal Netherlands Academy of Arts and Sciences in Amsterdam presented him with the Leeuwenhoek Medal, named after Antonie van Leeuwenhoek, who, by playing around with magnifying lenses, was the first person to observe bacteria swimming and growing in water. The medal was given only once in a decade for truly seminal contributions to science, and the previous recipients included none other than Louis Pasteur.

In 1922, d'Hérelle saved a thirty-two-year-old woman from cholecystitis—an infection of the gallbladder, from which she suffered for six months. Hospitalized with persistent high fevers, she had been so exhausted from the battle that doctors feared she was going to die. Finally, they decided to try a phage. From the sample of her gastric juices, d'Hérelle isolated the causative bacteria—a strain of E. coli—and cultivated a phage that preyed on it. Unlike the intestines, gallbladders aren't easily reachable for phages, so d'Hérelle injected his brew under her skin, hoping that the phages would make it into her bloodstream and ultimately arrive at the site of the infection. He was right. The phages found their food. The woman reacted with a spiking fever, but two hours later, her temperature dropped and stayed normal. "Eleven days later she went home completely healthy," d'Hérelle wrote in his notes, adding that other doctors began to adopt his method.[15] Now he knew he could use phages to treat internal organs, a useful fact since he was working on his next book, Les defenses de l'organisme, published in 1923.[16]

Soon after, the money at the Institute of Tropical Medicine began to dry up, and d'Hérelle was forced to look for another position. He sailed off to Alexandria for a job as laboratory chief, tasked with diagnosing and treating diseases on the ships passing through the Suez Canal[17] to prevent contagion between Asia and Europe. There, his dysentery phages became a standard treatment,[18] but the plague cases of the summer of 1925 propelled his reputation to new heights.

The phages he had long ago isolated from rat feces in remote

Indian villages finally proved their worth. And now the whole world wanted them. Yet not everyone—not even seasoned microbiologists sometimes—could make them work. Just like any living creatures, phages had their own whims, dietary preferences, and comfort zones. If conditions weren't right, they wouldn't perform.

In early 1926, a few months after his bubonic plague cure, d'Hérelle received a note from the Haffkine Institute in Bombay. The institute requested a "supply of remedy for trial in India under laboratory control."[19] D'Hérelle obliged, and the anti-plague phages arrived at Haffkine in March. But the same phages that so marvelously dissolved *Y. pestis* in Egypt would not do so in India. They grew slowly and took too long to lyse the cultures. D'Hérelle asked for an unpaid leave of absence from Alexandria and sailed off to Bombay to straighten out his misbehaving medicines.[20]

The problem lay not in science but in cultural details—namely, religious traditions and practices.

In order to grow the enteric bacteria—those that live or invade the intestines of animals or humans—in lab conditions, scientists commonly used the so-called Martin's medium, developed at the Pasteur Institute. This medium was essentially the classic meat broth, made from beef muscle and pig stomach—two ingredients widely used in European cuisine. In India, however, both components were impractical because they offended nearly everyone: Hindus couldn't use beef, and Muslims wouldn't touch pork. To solve this problem, scientists at the Haffkine Institute had long ago modified Martin's recipe, swapping the problematic proteins for an acceptable alternative: goat. They treated the goat tissues with hydrochloric acid to start the digestion (the acid normally present in the intestines that breaks down food), which typically made the enteric bacteria quite at home, so they reproduced and prospered. The scientists used the same medium for *Y. pestis*, but d'Hérelle's phages didn't like that combination and failed to act.

After playing around with the soup ingredients, d'Hérelle added another modification to the Martin's medium. He replaced the hydrochloric acid with papaya juice, which contains a natural digestive enzyme called *papain*. Phages liked that combination much better. D'Hérelle also improved Haffkine's filtration process for extracting the creatures from the papaya-goat blend—and out came perfectly virulent plague bacteria eaters.[21]

The reputations of d'Hérelle and his phages were restored, but that occurrence had clearly showed how finicky the living medicines were. Developing them at the level of mass production would require immense precision and strict attention to detail.

IN PARIS AGAIN

In early 1925, the three Eliavas boarded the train to Moscow, where they would change for another train—to Paris through Berlin. For Gogi and Amelia, this trip might as well have been their belated honeymoon; for Ganna, it was her first voyage to Europe since she was a baby. They traveled light, with minimal luggage, planning to fully update their wardrobes in Paris. The journey was supposed to be uneventful, but as often occurred in Gogi's peripatetic life, the trip soon took a detour.

Within a few hours, the train stopped in Baku, the capital of the Azerbaijan Republic on the Caspian Sea, and Gogi decided to take a walk to the seashore. Afraid that her excitable and easily distracted husband would lose track of time and miss the train, Amelia ventured out with him, leaving Ganna in their compartment. Her well-intended measure had the opposite effect: they both missed the train, which promptly whisked away their twelve-year-old daughter, along with all their documents, money, and luggage.

A car chase ensued. The panicked parents managed to find a

car and talk the driver into a train pursuit—a near-impossible feat for the 1920s when vehicles in the Soviet Union were rare. The train's next stop was the small town of Baladjari, a drive that would take about twenty minutes today. Luckily, trains traveled at a low speed on that particular stretch of railroad, so catching up with the locomotive was a distant possibility. The driver floored the pedal and gave chase. The Baladjari stop was supposed to be a quick one, but the passengers summoned the train crew to hold the departure. Glued to the windows as the train entered the station, the passengers watched for the cars on the road, which ran parallel to the tracks—until they spotted the crazily speeding one. "When I finally saw them getting out of the car and rushing to the train, my panic was replaced by anger," Ganna recalled. "How could you leave me?" she screamed at her parents, worming out of their hugs and ignoring their apologies.

In Moscow, the family spent two weeks dealing with what Gogi called "the formalities"—passports, papers, money. Ganna found Moscow disappointing. Compared to the clean and elegant Tbilisi, the capital of the socialist state resembled a huge village, unkempt and messy. The historical prerevolution capital was St. Petersburg, so Moscow still had years to catch up in everything from architecture to charm. After all the formalities were handled, Gogi had enough petty cash left over to make it to Paris, where a money transfer would be waiting.

To the family's horror, it wasn't. When the Eliavas arrived at the Parisian bank for their check, Gogi was told that no transfer had been received in his name yet. "Try again in a couple of weeks," said the clerk. By then, they would have run out of both money and clothes. Furious, Gogi left the bank, bent down to tie a shoe, and his only pair of trousers ripped at the seam. "And then a miracle happened," Ganna recalled. By an incredible coincidence—or perhaps thanks to Eliava's seemingly bottomless luck—his childhood friend from Batumi, a prosperous financier and the bank's employee, was passing by. "Gogi, I can't believe it. What brings you here?" he said with an embrace—and minutes later, the bank extended Eliava enough credit to last until the wire transfer came through.

Within a couple of days, the family settled in a three-room furnished apartment on a small street in a working-class neighborhood, where they stayed for the duration. With new clothes and a place to hang them, Gogi dove into his scientific work, passionately familiarizing himself with all the new achievements in microbiology that had developed during his four years of absence. His Pasteur colleagues welcomed him and his family with open arms. Pozerski, who enjoyed a reputation of a professional chef, having published cookbooks on the art and science of food making, immediately invited them for a posh dinner party; Eliava, not surprisingly, failed to arrive on time. "I'm glad Gogi is still true to himself," Pozerski humorously greeted the Eliavas as he opened the door to usher them in. "Two hours late, to be exact."

Together with Pozerski and other Pasteur colleagues, Eliava resumed his bacteriophage research. By then, bacteriophages had finally earned their reputation as agents of immunity but left a range of scientific questions to answer. For example, phages worked extremely well inside human or animal intestines, arresting lethal diseases within hours. They were spectacular with yersinia buboes. But their curative powers were far less clear when it came to the systemic infections, such as sepsis. If it was possible to save people from shigella-caused dysentery by giving them phage drinks, would it be possible to save them from staphylococcus-caused sepsis by injecting a phage solution into their veins? Exactly how small were the "bacteriophage corpuscles"—the viral particles that in today's terminology we call *virions* or *capsids*? Could they travel and spread within the body? Those were the types of questions

Eliava tried to answer during his Paris visits (he came back one more time in 1930).

The question about using bacteriophages against systemic infections was perhaps the most alluring—if it worked, it offered a new treatment paradigm. Yet bacteriophages were tricky to evaluate with consistency. While they lysed bacteria incredibly well in laboratory dishes, they would completely fail to dissolve bacteria in the bloodstream of sick animals, leaving researchers puzzled. "The question of the behavior of the bacteriophage, already sufficiently complex in vitro, reaches the maximum complexity, when it comes to transposing the phenomenon of d'Hérelle into an organism in vivo," Eliava and Pozerski wrote, embarking on a new experiment. "Bacteriophage, a microbicidal agent with incomparable activity in vitro, seemed predestined to fight septic diseases . . . But in practice, there is a considerable discrepancy between the action of the lytic agent in vitro and its activity in vivo, especially when it comes to studying the behavior of *Bacteriophagum intestinale* outside its normal habitat—the intestines—and introducing it, for example, into the circulatory stream."[22]

By then, scientists already knew about the existence of red and white blood cells. They also knew that the latter, by being part of the immune system, would attack and destroy any foreign organisms they detected. Therefore, the two collaborators hypothesized that some of the blood cells must be either destroying or deactivating the phage corpuscles before they could lyse the germs. "To find the truth of this discrepancy between the action of bacteriophage *in vitro* and *in vivo*, we have directed our research to determine which of the constituents of the blood can prevent the free exercise of bacteriophages' lytic power," they wrote.[23]

Working with rabbits and guinea pigs injected and sick with shigella, *E. coli*, and *S. aureus*, the collaborators tried to cure them by administering phages intravenously. That didn't work, except when the bacteria and the phages were given together in one injection, leading the duo to believe that the phages probably lysed the germs before they got fully annihilated by the blood cells. Eliava and Pozerski staged more experiments to determine exactly which cells were at fault and determined them to be the leukocytes—the white blood cells. "The insufficient action of the bacteriophage after its introduction into the circulatory stream would be due to the effective fixing of the bacteriophage corpuscles by the leukocytes," they wrote in their joint paper "On the Subject of Bacteriophage Adsorption by Leukocytes." "It is likely that subsequently, after fixation, the leukocytes destroy the bacteriophage."[24] Today, we know that bacteriophages are also filtered out of the blood by the liver and spleen.

Together with colleagues, Eliava tried to determine the size of the bacteriophage corpuscles—the virions or capsids. By squeezing phage solutions through increasingly fine filters, they estimated the corpuscles to be smaller than five micrometers.[25] Technically speaking they were correct, but not exactly precise—today, we measure phage sizes in nanometers (one thousand times smaller than a micrometer), with most of them ranging from twenty-four to two hundred nanometers in length.[26] Yet with their limited equipment and no electron microscopy, their conclusions were remarkable. Equally impressive were their experiments aimed to determine whether bacteriophages could penetrate the placenta, which typically serves as an impermeable barrier for foreign organisms, protecting the fetus. To answer that question, the collaborators gave pregnant guinea pigs bacteriophage injections, later drawing blood from them and—separately—from their fetuses inside the placenta. The guinea pigs' blood had a certain level of bactericidal activity—it killed or arrested germ growth in petri dishes. The fetal blood didn't, which led the collaborators to conclude that the phages couldn't cross over. "Thus, the placenta stops the bacteriophage," they wrote. "It presents an insurmountable

obstacle to the corpuscle."[27] (To some degree, this finding contradicted the fact that phages were being destroyed by the leukocytes,
but perhaps some still survived, just not in large enough numbers
to stop an acute sepsis within an animal.) Ultimately, Eliava suggested that the placental "plasmodium" behaves similar to a living
membrane, whose permeability certainly depends on numerous
and complex conditions, not just the particle size.[28] Notably, today's scientists are still researching the placenta permeability question.

As always, Eliava kept a wide circle of friends and colleagues.
He had worked with Charles Nicolle, who won a 1903 Nobel Prize
in medicine for discovering that typhus is spread by lice. He became a close friend of Eugène and Elisabeth Wollman, the found-
ing couple of the field we now call molecular genetics.[29] He even
made good friends with Calmette—d'Hérelle's earlier nemesis.
Eliava's research trip was supposed to take six months, but as he
grew absorbed in research, he needed more time to finish the experiments, so Calmette wrote a letter to the Georgian authorities
requesting to extend his stay, which was granted.[30]

In Paris, Eliava also grew close with his fellow Georgians, including Budu Mdivani—once the Red Army commissar whose
troops Ganna had watched marching into Tiflis in 1921, and now
a trade representative to France.[31] At his core, Gogi remained
deeply devoted to his Georgian roots, despite the glamour of his
Parisian life. He turned down an offer to work permanently at the
Pasteur Institute, with a famous reply: "Georgia needs me!" And
it did need him urgently. In his home state, people were still dying
from lack of medicine, shortage of vaccines, and a dearth of doctors. "He was a patriot of his nation," Devdariani-Malieva says of
her grandfather. "Not of the Soviet power, the true nature of which
he clearly saw as a smart and intellectual person—but of Georgia
and Georgian people."

After spending two years in Paris, Eliava headed home with forty boxes of medicines. True to character, he nearly missed the train, showing up five minutes before departure with all the containers in tow. Smuggled within them were "illegal gifts" for the women workers of the Bacteriological Institute—the much-coveted French perfume Chanel. The Soviet Union considered such vanity items a habit of the Western bourgeoisie and completely inappropriate for the new socialist society. Gogi, who was never good at taking no for an answer, shrugged off the rules. To trick the customs officials, who would surely poke through the contents of the boxes, he filled a bunch of ampoules with Chanel and sealed them to look like medicine. Lucky as always, he brought all of them to Tiflis without a hitch.

He still had about ten years of that luck ahead of him.

THE PHAGE BLOSSOM

The fateful year of 1925 propelled phages to their fame in more ways than one. Not only did d'Hérelle cure plague, but American author Sinclair Lewis published his novel *Arrowsmith*. A precursor to the modern science-fiction genre, it featured a young scientist, Martin Arrowsmith, who stumbles upon the phages' handiwork with uncanny similarity to d'Hérelle and, to some extent, Eliava. Like the inquisitive Georgian, Arrowsmith leaves a flask of murky, bacteria-laden water in his Rockefeller Institute lab and goes home to have dinner with his wife, Leora. When he returns hours later, he finds that all the bugs are gone. "I've got it!" he tells Leora, naming his newfound killer agent the X Principle. "I found something that eats bugs . . . dissolves them, kills them. May be a big new step in therapeutics." The institute puts out a proud press release—only to learn that a French scientist named d'Hérelle had just published a paper in *Comptes Rendus*, reporting that exact phenomenon, now named the bacteriophage—a plot twist that mirrors d'Hérelle's own experience with Twort's report.

Despite his disappointment, Arrowsmith soon gets a chance to test his phages against the bubonic plague killing thousands on St. Hubert, a fictional tropical island. Arrowsmith and Leora take off to start the rigorous trials on the island. He leaves Leora in "a safe spot" while he goes to conduct the trials in the epicenter of disease, but she contracts the plague in a lab accident, dying before Arrowsmith returns. The novel won the Pulitzer Prize and within a few years became a widely popular movie. Even more impressively, the novel actually foretold the future, to an extent—because it came out *before* d'Hérelle cured the plague-stricken youths. D'Hérelle must have read the book in early spring of 1925, a few months before he had a chance to put his plague phages to the test. He found it delightful and in March 1925 wrote about it to a friend: "Have you seen the novel Arrowsmith by Sinclair Lewis? It is rather entertaining since it is about almost entirely based on bacteriophage."[32]

There was a curious backstory to how the novel turned out to be so true to real science. Lewis worked closely with Paul de Kruif, a scientist turned science writer. A bacteriologist by education, de Kruif had worked at the Pasteur Institute during the war, at the same time as d'Hérelle. It's not clear whether the two ever worked together, but with all the controversy surrounding d'Hérelle's bacteria eaters, de Kruif was privy to the juicy details of the discovery and debates. After the war, de Kruif did his PhD at the lab of Frederick Novy at the University of Michigan, which became, perhaps not surprisingly, the first American institution to study bacteriophages—Novy imported a batch from d'Hérelle as early as 1921. In the meantime, de Kruif became a postdoctoral fellow at the Rockefeller Institute in New York, but grew dissatisfied with research and switched to science journalism, writing everything from explainers to exposés. Lewis and de Kruif met just as Lewis was pondering the subject for his new novel, and the two became friends. In 1923, while traveling in the Caribbean together, they outlined the novel's plot. Two years later, the phages "spilled out" of the white tower of scientific research and into the masses.[33]

To the general public, the fact that tiny creatures invisible even under the strongest microscopes possessed the ability to destroy the worst pathogens that afflicted humans was thrilling. It also brought immense hope that the era of infectious scourges might be nearing its end and that deadly epidemics could be stopped. Two months after d'Hérelle cured his four plague patients, *The New York Times* ran a story titled "Tiny and Deadly Bacillus Has Enemies Still Smaller." "What is the smallest living being? The microbe? Microbes have lesser microbes that prey upon them," the article said. "These lesser microbes have been named by their discoverer bacteriophages. They are so minute that the strongest microscope gives no indication of their presence."[34]

The article went on to explain how bacteriophages were serendipitously discovered and how, as parasites, they attack bacteria from the inside. "The victim bacillus swells up, becomes spherical in shape and finally explodes, liberating the parasites which have developed in its interior."[35] This powerful image—so far known only to the few people in research and now so picturesquely described by the top American newspaper to the general public—had a massive impact.

Word spread quickly and other scientists jumped on the phage train, experimenting successfully with the invisible microbe-slayers. Brazilian medics adopted phage therapy as a standard practice for treating dysentery even before d'Hérelle's spectacular feat. Epidemiologist J. da Costa Cruz at the Oswaldo Cruz Institute in Rio de Janeiro prepared ten thousand ampoules of dysentery phages and sent them to hospitals and clinics across Brazil. The physicians were in awe of how quickly their patients bounced back—usually in a day or two. They marveled at the fact that phages had no side effects. "Doses of bacteriophage as great as 4 c.c. could be given subcutaneously or intramuscularly without more reaction than would accompany the administration of a similar amount of saline—that is a slightly sore arm. That is the first respect in which bacteriophage lysed cultures differ from the usual vaccine. In about 200 injections I have not had a single reaction."[36]

Industry jumped on the opportunity—with mixed results that would have long-term consequences for phage science and therapy. Several American companies began to manufacture phage preparations. E. R. Squibb and Sons sold staphylococcus bacteriophage in twenty-milliliter vials for $3.50, which promised to work for a range of staph skin infections that caused painful boils, claiming an almost immediate pain-relieving effect. Lilly Research Laboratories advertised "bacterial antigens in a Water Soluble Jelly Base . . . for local applications in the treatment of certain infections." Called Staphylo-Jel, it pledged to work fast, liquify "necrotic core," and cause little scarring. The Swan-Myers division of Abbott Laboratories also marketed bacteriophage preparations for staph infections.[37] European companies followed suit. Berlin-based Antipiol sold Enterofagos for multiple intestinal diseases.[38] The German Bacteriophage Society began selling phages for *E. coli* and staph in dry form, as tablets.[39]

Phage medicines were deceptively easy to produce. It seemed that anyone with a few vials of dirty water could make them. Just boil some meat scraps, feed them to your target bacteria, and then transfer that brew to the phages that you fished out of the nearest sewage gutter. That misleading assumption, with no regulatory oversight, resulted in many concoctions that either worked poorly or didn't work at all. Moreover, some of these amateur phage-makers were either ignorant or unscrupulous enough that they sold their so-called cures to treat diseases caused not by bacteria but by entirely different organisms, such as fungi, parasites, or viruses. One company promised to treat hives, eczema, and herpes. Needless to say, phages did nothing for those, undermining people's trust, d'Hérelle's reputation, and the general belief in his therapy.

That pushed d'Hérelle to create his own Laboratoire du Bactériophage in Paris, which began growing living medicines for dysentery, *E.coli*, skin infections, and more. The lab was a family endeavor.[40] D'Hérelle's younger daughter, Huberte—the one before whose birthday the bacteriophage was named—married a man named Theodore Mazure, who became an assistant at the lab, taking the reins when his commonly absentee father-in-law was globetrotting.[41] The advertising pamphlet read, "When prescribing bacteriophages specify Bacteriophage d'Herelle, THE ORIGINAL BACTERIOPHAGE," likely to indicate that the medicine was indeed of a trustworthy quality. Apparently, d'Hérelle sought no profit from the enterprise, investing all proceeds in research.[42]

In 1926, he published his next book, *The Bacteriophage and Its Behavior*, in which he focused on proving that bacteriophages were living creatures by articulating their ability to assimilate and adapt to the bacteria they attack. Like his previous work, this volume was also promptly translated into English by the same George H. Smith of the Yale University School of Medicine. Despite some readers wanting better proof that phages were alive—they noted that, unlike most beings, phages didn't seem to respire, because they didn't produce any measurable carbon dioxide[43]—overall, d'Hérelle's new work was well received. With several books to his name, a list of papers, and cohorts of patients cured from the worst infectious scourges, he finally found long-overdue acceptance.

The American scientific establishment welcomed him with

open arms. In 1928, Yale University offered him a professorship and a sizable three-year budget, with a promise to readjust it to fit his needs afterward. "Famous scientist appointed to faculty of the Yale School of Medicine," read the press release when d'Hérelle accepted. That offer also included a laboratory space and considerable prestige—everything that d'Hérelle always dreamed of achieving. But paradoxically, instead of throwing himself into his new position, he spent a lot of his time away from it. By the late 1920s, he was so frequently invited to deliver lectures within American research circles that he spent more time talking about science than actually doing it—at least from the perspective of Yale's leadership. He was nearly four months late to start his first year at Yale because he had traveled all over California and the West Coast, arriving in October instead of July. And then he was off to Philadelphia and later to California again. Notably, these engagements resulted not only in fame but generous honorariums.[44]

His launch of the Laboratoire du Bactériophage also coincided with Yale's offer and, in a way, clashed with it. He came to Yale to do mostly fundamental research, yet by now he wanted to focus on making his medicines available to people. Stretching himself thin between two continents proved difficult. Research obligations necessitated his presence at Yale. The fledgling enterprise demanded his attention in Paris. Without informing the Yale dean of his "side business," d'Hérelle took extended summer vacations in France or requested urgent leaves of absence. Over the five years that he stayed with the university, the tensions between the wayward professor and the school's leadership simmered slowly, culminating when d'Hérelle delivered his resignation in 1933, just as the Great Depression engulfed the country.[45]

He had a better place to go and better prospects to look forward to. He was off to Tiflis.

5

Together in Tiflis

"Mirra, do you have lunch?" Gogi called, rushing in through the front door. "I'm starving!"

This was a rhetorical question. Of course there was lunch. The Eliava's family cook—an elderly woman who couldn't read or write but remembered the abolition of serfdom in 1861—lived with the family like a babushka, a grandmother. But what Gogi was really asking was whether there would be dessert at the end of the meal. The answer was also yes—purchased from his favorite bakery nearby. He needed that sugar fix to get through the rest of the day. The construction of two new floors at the Bacteriological Institute's main building had ground to a halt because there was not enough cement, sawed wood, and roof tiles. And that was only part of a larger problem.

While Mirra and the babushka set the table, Gogi collapsed onto the sofa, exhausted from yet another chaotic morning.[1] All of his days were spent in constant motion, presenting, convincing, persuading, and running from place to place. At Gogi's brisk walking pace, the Machabeli building was only five minutes away from his house on Shio Chitadze Street,[2] but by the early 1930s, the institute's departments were scattered over multiple locations, so he was constantly rushing between them. The Pasteur Department that gave rabies shots was on Technical Street, the lab producing smallpox medicines on Tatianovskaya, the Epidemiological Department was part of a hospital in the Avlabari neighborhood, and the Sera Department was out on the outskirts in Saburtalo, on the Mtkvari's banks.

And then there was teaching. By this time, Eliava held a professorship at the Tiflis Medical University. He headed the university's Microbiology Department. He was the chairman of its Hygiene Department. He taught classes to students and practicing physicians. And between all that, he found a few minutes to stage lab experiments, but rarely the time to write them down for a journal paper—a sore point for Amelia, who begged him to focus more on science than daily minutiae. "Why are you wasting your gift of research?" she prodded. "I have to get things moving," he would respond. He often had to be in several places at once, so he was now asking his superiors to buy his institute a Ford truck.[3]

After lunch, he'd take a quick nap, until Zitka, the family's terrier, would wake him up by licking his face, as if signaling it was time to go. "This dog is so smart, I swear it will talk to me one day," he would say, playing with her for a few minutes before he took off. He had no answer when Amelia asked what time he would return home. In addition to the daily grind, he had to write a detailed memo to the People's Commissariat listing all the issues imperiling the institute's work for the past few months—starting with the misappropriated brick wall. He had too many holes to plug, sometimes quite literally.

The institute's Saburtalo location that housed stables and labs had lost part of its fence. Initially built to surround the thirteen hectares allocated to the campus, part of the half-mile wall was demolished the previous year. The Tiflis Council decreed that the local community needed the bricks more than the institute, so they had been promptly reallocated, leaving a gaping hole. The issue wasn't the aesthetic but the fact that it allowed strangers to wander around the labs that dealt with infectious agents. And then there was a "reverse-contamination" danger. Attracted by the lush green lawns of the institute's grounds, the cattle from neighboring villages came to graze on the grass, bringing a variety of microorganisms on their bodies and in their manure.[4]

"The institute's territory is completely open from one side, which made it accessible for cattle that may be infected with various diseases and may transfer them to experimental animals," Eliava wrote in a desperate letter to Petre Aghniashvili at the Georgian People's Commissariat on November 1, 1932. "Additionally, strangers are entering the territory. It is imperative to urgently restore the isolation barrier. If the executive committee (EC) is unable to implement this task, the institute is ready to cover the expenses, but in this case the EC should take a responsibility to provide 250000 bricks immediately."[5]

Even more damaging was the shortage of oats, barley, and hay, which directly affected the production of medicines. To make enough vaccines and serums to neutralize bacteria and their toxins, the institute housed 90 horses that generated therapeutic compounds to be extracted from their blood. Humans who give blood must be well nourished, and so must the equine donors, who need nutritious oats and barley. But the horses—in addition to the institute's 1,200 rabbits, 600 guinea pigs, and numerous rats, mice, and pigeons—weren't getting their feed regularly from the governing authorities. The existing laws prioritized feeding the Red Army horses before all other animals, so when food was scarce, the institute had to fend for itself. To keep the animals healthy, the institute needed fifteen tons of oats and twenty tons of hay a month, but in 1932, it was barely getting any.[6]

"During the last two months, only due to extraordinary efforts, did the institute manage to get two tons of barley and five tons of oats," Eliava wrote. "The horses that are the valuable producers of sera, whose immunized blood is used as a source of sera, were fed surrogate, such as bran only. The starving animals couldn't survive donating blood on this feed—and died." The institute—now charged with supplying vaccines and medicines to the neighboring republics of Armenia and Turkmenistan, and even to Moscow and Leningrad, whose own labs sometimes couldn't produce enough—was struggling to fulfill requests.[7]

"If the above-mentioned needs are not satisfied, the institute will not be able to cope with the increasing demands. It was already unable to provide anti-typhoid vaccine for the existing epidemic of typhoid fever, and it will not be able to meet the full production volume expected from it," Eliava stressed, arguing that the laws must grant the institute's animals the same priority as the military horses, if not more. At the end of his memo, he also requested 250 meters of roofing iron, 12,000 roof tiles, 12 iron beams, plus truckloads of cement and wood to finish the Machabeli additions.[8] His plea worked. Within two weeks, Aghniashvili at the People's Commissariat approved nearly all the requests. The fact that Stalin himself was a Georgian and was willing to throw money at his home state might have helped the cash flow.

The holes, including the one that compromised the wall, would be plugged, but Eliava couldn't stop. He had plans for a much bigger future for his brainchild. He imagined it as an international bacteriophage research, manufacturing, and treatment facility. But to accomplish this goal, he needed help. And he knew just the right person to partner with: the father of bacteriophages.

TOGETHER IN TIFLIS

After attending the Congress on Immunology of the Royal Academy of Italy in Rome, d'Hérelle headed to Tiflis in September 1933 with his wife, Marie. By then, their children had long grown up, and the d'Hérelles were empty nesters.[9] The lengthy sea voyage from Marseille across the Mediterranean, the Dardanelles, the Bosporus, and finally the Black Sea took them over a month—but d'Hérelle was looking forward to the Tiflis promise.[10]

The aging scientist was eager to start using phages on a larger scale—in clinical trials and in the actual clinics. His Paris laboratory was already producing several types of living medicines named after the germs they destroyed— Bacté-coli-phage, Bacté-staphy-phage, and Bacté-intesti-phage, among others.[11] But an institutional backing, especially at the level of Eliava's offer, would make a major difference. Eliava granted d'Hérelle a spacious laboratory to do research. He had hired and trained several young lab assistants, recent graduates of the Tiflis University, who were now ready to work with the famed bacteriophagist. But even more importantly, Eliava was going to plug d'Hérelle into a vast network of practicing doctors, with whom the French scientist could collaborate to make his living medicines widely available to people. Eliava's grand visions for the Bacteriophage Institute—an establishment focused specifically on bacteriophages—promised to bring d'Hérelle's lifelong vision to fruition.

The d'Hérelles arrived in Batumi in October, greeted by Eliava's hearty embraces and heaps of flowers.[12] To assure his guests wanted for nothing, he procured a car and a personal chauffeur for their use. D'Hérelle settled in the Hotel Oriant on Shota Rustaveli Avenue,[13] not far from Machabeli Street, and threw himself into the research. He brought with him expensive laboratory equipment, including a wooden desk and a handsome incubating cabinet with carved wooden doors that kept the cultures at about 37°C (98.6°F).

Consumed by the goal of cultivating highly efficient bacteriophages that could consistently and reliably stop infections,[14] d'Hérelle was documenting the process in minute detail. Having run his Paris lab for about five years now, he had amassed a great deal of knowledge he could now put to practice. As he tested his bacteria eaters, he wrote guidelines for Eliava and his laboratory staff, training them on everything he knew.

He laid out clear instructions where in nature medics should be looking to find bacteriophages for treatments: in the intersection of rivers and sewage. Yet, he cautioned, not all bacteriophages were easily found there at all times. While phages for dysentery and cholera could be isolated from wastewater nearly daily, others, like staphylococcus and streptococcus, were apparently seasonal, appearing only during certain months a year. "Since 1928, my assistants in the Paris laboratory isolated numerous bacteriophages by sampling the wastewaters weekly," he noted. "They found that bacteriophages against streptococcus can be isolated only in summer between the months of May and August. Isolating them during other times of the year is a rare occurrence, which probably has to do with seasonal diseases caused by these microorganisms." He acknowledged that he still hadn't been able to isolate bacteriophages against several bacterial pathogens—for example, the gonorrhea-causing gonococcus. He concluded that those phages were remarkably rare but remained convinced that they existed; otherwise, the germs would uncontrollably proliferate in the world.

To achieve mass production, these isolated phages had to be grown in large amounts, which d'Hérelle knew from his own experience in Bombay and elsewhere was no easy feat. Over time, d'Hérelle developed precise recipes for growing living medicines, which he taught to his assistants in Tiflis. He suggested mixing five hundred grams of finely minced beef or lamb with two hundred cubic centimeters of water and leaving it overnight. In the morning, he recommended squeezing one hundred cubic centimeters of the resulting "meat juice" and adding five grams of salt. To that brew, he instructed the lab to add nine hundred cubic centimeters of sewage water and ten cubic centimeters of bacterial culture, for which the bacteriophage was to be isolated. "Then place the culture to incubate for 24 hours and pass it through the Chamberland filter,"[15] he wrote. "The bacteriophage in question will be in your filtrate."

That wasn't the end of the cultivating process—far from it. The resulting bacteriophage, whether for cholera, dysentery, or staph, wouldn't necessarily perform at its best right from the start. It could be a weak bacteriophage, d'Hérelle cautioned. Therefore, its potency, or virulence, against the specific bacterial strain had to be improved. D'Hérelle took great care in explaining how to cultivate these more aggressive bacteriophages. He called them "bacteriophage races," using the term *race* the same way scientists use the term *strain* when speaking about bacteria.[16] Essentially, he was cultivating specific bacteriophage races to attack specific bacterial strains.

The process, once again, had to do with the nature of all living creatures. Just like any beings, phages adapted to their environment and their food sources. D'Hérelle had long ago noticed that phages that weren't particularly active against certain strains—of, for example, shigella—would become more aggressive after being passed through several shigella cultures because they would adapt to prey on it better. So d'Hérelle developed a method of "training" phages on the desired strains.

"This process is very simple," he wrote with his typical confidence. "The bacteria should be seeded into a bouillon-containing tube, which then should be immediately inoculated with a drop of filtrate containing a weak bacteriophage. After 24 hours of incubating, the liquid should be passed through the Chamberland filter and this newly obtained bacteriophage filtrate should be used to repeat the procedure. That same process should be repeated 10 to

20 times." The number of repetitions, however, wasn't set in stone, he noted, because as living entities, bacteriophages had minds of their own. Unlike the molecules of antibiotics that always worked the same way—until they would stop working—phages operated with their own speed and aptitude. "The ability to adapt to new bacterial cultures varies greatly between different bacteriophage races," d'Hérelle noted. "Some races, very weak at onset of the procedure, can reach their maximum level of virulence only after several passages. Others, despite being more potent in the beginning, don't necessarily increase their virulence even after many passages."

Although he described it as simple, the procedure required concentrated manual work, precision, and time. If every filtrate had to incubate for twenty-four hours, the desired bacteriophage race would take ten to twenty days to obtain. Moreover, that time could vary, and the resulting bacteriophage could still perform weaker than desired.

Evolution also could derail a phage result. Sometimes phages wouldn't be able to extinguish all bacteria in a sample, because a few bugs would become resistant. In those cases, phages couldn't stick to their surface or penetrate their walls with their tails—the molecular lock-and-key structures wouldn't match up. Sometimes phages wouldn't be able to successfully reproduce inside the bugs. The resistant population would grow, making the once nearly clear solution cloudy again—which, inside a human being, would be bad news. Inside a flask, that meant that the lab had to go phage-hunting again. Eliava and his lab assistants would travel to the spots where wastewater effluent flowed into the river and plunge their buckets in, hoping to fish out better phages.

With such complexity and seemingly infinite variability, it was no wonder that d'Hérelle worked long hours, pipetting, filtrating, and incubating day in and day out. "His drive stemmed from his absolute confidence that bacteriophages would save humankind from infections," recalled Elena Makashvili, Eliava's assistant and lab technician who learned the process from d'Hérelle and later directed the institute's bacteriophage department. "Day after day, he worked on bacteriophages lysing *Staphylococcus aureus*, *Shigella dysenteriae*, *Vibrio cholerae* and *Bacillus pestis*."[17]

The detailed instructions he was putting together were meant to become the guidebook for the bacteriophage manufacturing plant that Eliava and d'Hérelle envisioned building in the near future. As soon as they were ready, Eliava would petition the People's Commissariat for the funds. In the meantime, the two collaborators worked on "advertising" phage therapeutics they had in the pipeline. Eliava, a lecturer himself, had brought his friend over not only as a research scientist but as a professor at the school for continuing education of physicians,[18] who were eager to battle diseases that regularly took their patients' lives.

Two opposing personalities—one serious and proper, the other gregarious and mischievous—d'Hérelle and Eliava complemented each other, which is likely what made their partnership so successful. Together, they prepared lectures, taught classes, and worked with medics to disseminate the knowledge about phage biology and therapy, broadcasting their ideas to a wide audience of receptive listeners. The move proved brilliant because it assured the future survival of phage therapy. In the hands of practicing physicians, d'Hérelle's living medicines sprouted such remarkably strong roots in Georgia and beyond that they remained official treatments even after antibiotics became dominant. Alexander Tsulukidze, professor of general surgery at Tiflis Medical Institute, had fully adapted them in his medical practice, publishing fourteen papers between 1935 and 1957.[19]

As the cold weather arrived later in late 1933, d'Hérelle developed bronchitis, but that didn't stop him from going to the lab, not for a single day. He was very unhappy if even a minute of his time was wasted on something not connected with microbiology. "He was in by eight o'clock in the morning and stayed long hours," recalled Irakli Georgadze, another lab technician who worked with d'Hérelle and later became the institute's director. "We, the young laboratory hands, had trouble catching up with him." The French scientist also impressed his staff with his universal skills. "He was a virtuoso when it came to lab work and could do absolutely everything. Once, when one of us forgot to sterilize the next batch of specialized pipettes, he took a regular glass pipette, sat down at the burner and, like a professional glassblower, blew the pipette he needed," Georgadze wrote years later. That glass-blowing trick blew their mind. "We were endlessly surprised by him."[20]

The staff also marveled at the precision with which d'Hérelle worked and how accurately he understood the inner workings of the microbial mechanisms with the imperfect imaging tools he had. "He didn't have the electronic microscopes at his disposal, but his ideas about the phage's invasion into a bacterial cell were astonishingly precise," Georgadze said. "Accuracy was his main characteristic. He was extremely so. In his experiments. In his relationships with his colleagues."[21] In everything.

It was Eliava who occasionally poked at his friend's exactitude with a prank or a trick. One of them became a family legend, shares Dimitry Devdariani, who heard the story from his grandmother Ganna more than a few times. Frequent guests in Eliava's house, the d'Hérelles often joined them for dinner. One time when they came in, Eliava wasn't there. "Gogi will be a bit late, but I have a friend joining us today," Amelia announced, introducing them to an eccentric and flamboyant guest. The woman, wearing a flashy dress, an ostentatious hat, high heels, and excessive makeup seemed to have immediately developed a brazen affection for d'Hérelle, flirting shamelessly, which annoyed and irritated Marie. The spectacle continued until the femme fatale lost all decency and attempted to sit herself on the Frenchman's knees. Marie turned red in the face, but before the situation escalated any further, the interloper ripped off her hat and wig, revealing—to the couple's utter surprise—the familiar haircut of their friend Gogi. "You can have him back," Gogi said to Marie with a smile so disarming that she couldn't bring herself to be angry with him. "I wasn't really going to take him from you."[22]

Gogi used his social talents for team-building events too. On holidays and weekends, he organized events and performances for his crew. "We often got together, singing, dancing, or staging little performances," recalled Nunu Gelasonidze, another lab technician. "Sometimes he invited actors. Sometimes he brought musicians. Sometimes he brought his wife and she would sing for us while he accompanied her on the piano. We were a great team, and we had a lot of fun, and Gogi was always the mastermind of everything."[23]

The institute's camaraderie coupled with the government's willingness to fund research left d'Hérelle enamored with the young Soviet state. He felt that "the era of unmatched development and blossom of science should launch in the Soviet Union" because the government put people and their health first. "Laboratories for biological research are opening everywhere in this humongous country, the scientific life is deepening and intensifying," he wrote, "contrary to the capitalist countries where it seems to be increasingly slowing down; there science was doomed to be the first victim of the global world economic crisis."[24]

The French scholar had been prescient in his visions of bacteriophage biology. But in his view of the Soviet Union, he was not.

THE TROUBLE BREWING BACKSTAGE

The Soviet dedication to science was indeed sincere, but behind this generous façade, trouble was brewing. The d'Hérelles arrived at Tiflis at a pivotal moment in Soviet politics. On one hand, the country appeared to be thriving. New cities were built, new factories erected, and new mines opened. On the other hand, much of this prosperity was achieved at the expense of everyday citizens. The new economic policies that ruthlessly imposed industrialization and pushed villages into collective farms were especially harmful to the same poor workers and peasants that the revolution had promised to defend. In Ukraine, where peasants traditionally owned small family farms and fought against collectivization, Stalin instituted Holodomor, a famine that killed millions. The massive construction of smelteries and hydroelectric stations, which demanded hard physical labor, worked their builders into the ground. Dreams for the new society were souring, overall morale was dipping, and Stalin began to worry about his grip on the country. One of his concerns was that, disillusioned with his rule, some border republics like Georgia or Ukraine could separate into independent nations.

Stalin's worries weren't unfounded. Ukraine and Georgia indeed had "nationalist clubs"—close circles of high officials who entertained the prospect of becoming sovereign states. These nationalist ideas were quite strong in Georgia, which had been independent for a short while before the Red Army annexed it over a decade prior. But if Georgia separated, it could be persuaded by hostile capitalist countries to allow foreign armies to enter its territory, which would leave the USSR vulnerable to attacks. Many European countries considered the Soviet Union a major threat to their way of life, so Stalin's fear of foreign invasions was real and amplified by his decreasing popularity. Nationalist thinking—as well as any real or perceived deviation from the Communist Party's line—had to be eradicated not only in Georgia but everywhere in the Soviet state. Dissent had to be extinguished before it could spread. The People's Commissariat for Internal Affairs, abbreviated as NKVD for Narodniy Komitet Vnutrennih Del, was charged with this task.

Historically, dissenters tended to be among the educated independent thinkers, who weren't afraid to speak up. Many of the intelligentsia—engineers, architects, doctors, scientists, and writers—had studied abroad, spent time in other countries, spoke multiple languages, had friends who were foreign nationals, and thus could be accused of being spies. It is among those circles that the NKVD was going to look the hardest for the "foreign elements" and "enemies of the people." One of the early alarming signs was a 1928 trial of fifty-three mining engineers from Shakhty (Mines) in the Rostov region, accused of sabotage and wrecking (destroying socialist property and achievements), and forced into confessions.[25] Each trial was reported in the press as a triumph over traitors and spies.

So far, Georgia managed to escape the worst of Stalin's terror—and there was a reason for that. In the early stages of the revolution, the Communist Party split into two camps: the Bolsheviks, from the word *bolshe* meaning "bigger" or "majority," and the Mensheviks, from the word *menshe*, as in "minority." The Bolsheviks believed that brute force exercised in establishing the dictatorship of the proletariat was justified by the greatness of the future society. The Mensheviks had more respect for human life and thought the same goals could be achieved with less bloodshed. The Soviet Georgian government was Menshevik-leaning. The two Georgian Red Army leaders Pilipe Makharadze and Budu Mdivani—who became Eliava's Parisian friend—were more humane than their brethren, reining in other parts of the Soviet State. At some point in the early 1920s, they even tried to revolt against the party's rule, but settled the conflict.[26]

But that was about to change. In fact, it was changing already—and soon would threaten Gogi, his work, and the future of his innovations.

THE BLOODSUCKER OF THE GEORGIAN PEOPLE

In the early 1930s, a new player, as vicious as he was clever, rose up the ranks in Georgian politics to eventually become Stalin's confidant and right-hand man. Lavrenti Beria would go down in history as one of the most feared leaders of the Soviet regime—a psychopath who enjoyed personally torturing his victims, and a sexual predator with whom Stalin wouldn't allow his own teenage daughter to be left alone.

An engineer by training, Beria made a spectacular career in politics, undeterred by moral qualms. Unlike the revolutionary leaders before him, he had no ideals, no principles, and no visions for the great society, other than establishing his own absolute control.[27] By 1931, he was the head of the Georgian secret police—the most vicious branch of the NKVD—and shortly after he became first secretary of the Georgian Party Central Committee, essentially consolidating his grip on both institutions. From 1933 to 1934, he was behind the first round of arrests that swept Georgia to "clean it from foreign elements," targeting veterinarians, agronomists, and engineers for alleged acts of economic sabotage on behalf of a counterrevolutionary Georgian National Center.[28]

An arrogant bully hungry for power, Beria demanded respect and reverence from the Georgian intelligentsia, but they weren't in any hurry to oblige. Eliava's circles in particular detested Beria. Gogi's friends were engineers, singers, artists, writers, and poets— well educated and freethinking. Beria, on the contrary, was neither well educated nor well read. He was rude, crude, and vulgar—and a womanizer whose wandering eyes often landed on the wives of his colleagues and acquaintances. He became obsessed with Tina-tin Jikia, a legendary blue-eyed beauty married to one of Eliava's best friends, Vladimir, an engineer building a hydroelectric station on the Rioni River in western Georgia. The couple lived down the block from Beria, which fueled his infatuation. On one occasion, having walked by the Jikias' place while they hosted a party, Beria sent an underling to order her to come to his house, but she re-fused, explaining that she was entertaining guests (one of whom openly cursed Beria).[29] Beria became so persistent and brazen in his overtures that at another social gathering, Vladimir publicly reprimanded him by recounting aloud an ancient fable, in which a shah's vizier killed his monarch for lusting over his wife.

Some legends purport that Beria cast his gaze on Amelia too, who remained a stunning woman with an incredible voice, even in her late forties. Although she had left the theater and struggled with polycythemia—a rare condition in which the body makes too many blood cells as it ages—she still performed in concerts and on the radio.[30] "She was too striking for Beria to miss," Nata-lia Devdariani-Malieva says, but "if he'd ever made a move, Gogi would kill him." Whether it was true or not, the animosity between Beria and Eliava seethed. A true patriot of Georgia who passed on the prestigious Pasteur Institute in order to heal and cure people of his home state, Eliava hated the ruthless, self-centered party ca-reerist paving his way to the top with the bodies of his fellow coun-tryfolk in his wake. And because Gogi did everything passionately, he hated Beria with a passion too, without ever bothering to hide it. "He was an absolute free spirit, who was never afraid of anything or anyone," Natalia says. "Definitely not Gogi." Not only did the two clash on multiple occasions, but Eliava openly scorned Beria more than once. Life presented him with plenty of occasions.

When Giorgi Balanchivadze—who later became the famed American choreographer George Balanchine—staged a new ballet at the Tiflis opera house celebrating Georgian culture, Beria banned it as too "nationalistic" and not "patriotically Soviet enough." The artistic community, among which Gogi had many friends, had relished the performance and was beyond disappointed, so he spared no strong opinions about Beria's cultural acumen. "Only an idiot and a moron who knows nothing about music and art could kill this brilliant performance."[31]

For one of his social gatherings, Gogi trained Zitka to turn away from a treat. "Beri, beri, beri," he would tell the terrier, waving a piece of sugar in front of her, which in Russian meant, "Take it, take it." When pronounced fast, it sounded just like the last name of the loathed party tycoon, so at the end of the trick, Gogi announced, "See, even the dog wants nothing to do with Beria. She turns away just at the mention of his name." In another show, Gogi wouldn't let Beria's car pass when the two of them met at an intersection—and crossed in front of him, which the mogul took as deep disrespect. But perhaps the most daring was the comment that Eliava once made to Beria's face.

Beria had been sick with a strange illness—a mild fever that wouldn't go away for days, leaving his physicians puzzled. Concerned, Beria had called for Eliava, who, in addition to his scientific work, had a reputation as a shrewd diagnostician. "When doctors couldn't establish a diagnosis, they called Gogi," says Devdariani-Malieva. "So Beria wanted him too."

Gogi showed up with a blood test kit. As he filled up the vials with Beria's blood, the party don made a joke. "Don't suck all the blood out of me!" Eliava's comeback left Beria white with rage.

"Why not?" Gogi responded. "You suck the blood of the entire nation. You're the bloodsucker of all the Georgian people."

Beria never forgot any snubs. Spiteful and vindictive, he collected these slights like ammunition until he could finally exact revenge on anyone who dared to offend him. In the spring of 1934, when d'Hérelle left for Paris for a few months and Eliava turned his full attention to building the Bacteriophage Institute, Beria got his first moment of satisfaction.

Eliava had big plans—he now envisioned a world-class Tiflis Bacteriophage Institute that would integrate a treatment center, an epidemiological station, a phage-growing plant, and a research facility. To begin, he was going to build the bacteriophage manufacturing facility.

The project required money, so Eliava submitted another detailed report (*dokladnaya zapiska*) to the SovNarKom. In the document, he explained the therapeutic potential of bacteriophages[32] and the need for an institution dedicated to the subject. He outlined the geographically wide and biologically diverse applications of phages, which made them invaluable medicines for many deadly diseases. He wrote about phages for dysentery, a common summer affliction. He wrote about phages for the bubonic plague. He wrote about phages' application for the diseases of war, such as typhoid and cholera, which took more lives than the actual fighting. He also stressed the phages' great potential for wound treatments, an unmatched healing paradigm in the pre-antibiotic era. He wrote that the most pressing move right now was building the manufacturing facility to grow phages not only for Georgia but for other republics and the military. And he praised the international reputation of d'Hérelle and the importance of his support for the project.[33]

Eliava was clever to hit on all the right points. Mass production of phage medicines would not only save civilian lives but give the Red Army a steep advantage over its adversaries, which was particularly appealing in the era of heightened invasion concerns.[34] Bringing a world-class scientist to the scene would also draw attention from abroad—the Soviet leaders craved international acclaim. Moreover, Eliava already had secured some money to start. Petre Aghniashvili—the man who had previously given him an uninterrupted supply of oats and barley—had committed to a sum of 200,000 rubles, but Eliava's estimates were just short of a million, at 940,000. He was now asking for the remainder.[35]

However, the person holding the purse strings this time was Beria. A shrewd politician keenly interested in his career, Beria must have realized the institute's promise—as an international establishment and the army's medical backbone, it would elevate his own persona in Stalin's eyes. But instead, or maybe despite the opportunity, Beria saw his chance to get even. Or perhaps he wanted to teach Eliava a lesson, proving his superiority. In either case, he dismissed the proposal with an expletive, which he reportedly wrote across the page.

It was clear that Eliava couldn't expect any local party support for his lifelong endeavor. But Gogi never took no for an answer. So he found other ways. He played smarter and he went higher. He simply bypassed Beria, going all the way to the top. With this dangerously bold move, which was typical of him, he sealed both the success of his institution and his own tragic fate.

THE BACTERIOPHAGE BIBLE

D'Hérelle returned in November 1934 with gifts for his lab personnel. "My dear Ellen," he told Elena Makashvili, presenting her with a fashionable French hat, "I think it will look great on you."[36] He and his wife found Tiflis even nicer than before—in just a few months, the city had gone through an impressive makeover.

The narrow, winding streets where a person and a donkey could barely pass each other were being widened and repaved. Renovated buildings shined with freshly painted façades. New stores and cafés dotted the streets. Even the city's name itself was about to be refreshed soon—changed to the more authentic version we use today: Tbilisi, from *tbili*, the warm springs. Marie d'Hérelle described these developments in her diary. "The new square is resplendent and surrounded by stores ... There are perfumeries, pretty pharmacies, cafes, a large ready to wear store for men. All the buildings have had a facelift which gives the city a nicer appearance than last year," she wrote. "So many changes! They have built beautiful quays along the Kura [Mtkvari] and a pretty promenade bordered by trees."[37] Stalin was throwing money at his home state, and overall, the Soviet Union seemed to be upholding its promise of a better, happier society.

The nationwide newspaper *Pravda*, or *Truth*, proudly covered the French scientist's arrival. "Professor d'Herelle is coming to the USSR for the second time," read the article that described him as "one of the most outstanding microbiologists in Western Europe."[38] D'Herelle's overall view of phages as living entities and their holistic role in human health had strong supporters among Soviet researchers. Sophia Kazarnovskaia at the Leningrad Pasteur Institute wrote that bacteriophage was a "substance with features of a creature."[39] The visionary earth scientist Vladimir Vernadsky considered bacteriophages to be the smallest and most liminal units of life. The scholars and their country appeared warm and welcoming, so d'Hérelle and Eliava traveled extensively, often as families. D'Hérelle, an amateur but capable shutterbug, indulged in photography, taking rolls of pictures—of cities, landscapes, people, and Gogi galloping along on his horse Infanta. The photos, along with the developed rolls, are still in the annals of the Pasteur Institute, and some are in Tbilisi.

The two collaborators attended microbiology conferences in Baku and Leningrad, speaking and presenting. They exchanged ideas and results with colleagues. They visited major research centers in Moscow and Kharkiv—a large Ukrainian city that also had a thriving bacteriophage research scene by that time. Scientists at the Kharkiv Mechnikov Institute of Microbiology and Immunology had been isolating and using phages to treat epidemics of scarlet fever, typhoid, and dysentery in Donbas, the pillar region of the Soviet industrialization because of its coal mines and heavy industry. Workers flocked to Donbas from all over the country, bringing their microbes with them, while the crowded conditions and poor hygiene made outbreaks inevitable. By 1929, the Kharkiv crew was using phages not only for treatment but even for prophylaxis of dysentery. The two bacteriophage teams, Georgian and Ukrainian, immediately struck up a collaboration, committing to exchange bacterial cultures and phages, as well as research plans and outcomes of treatments.[40]

While in Moscow, d'Hérelle met Grigory Kaminsky, the People's Commissar of Health for the Soviet Union, the country's highest wellness authority. Kaminsky invited him to do research in the capital, offering to devote an entire scientific institute to the study of phage therapy. D'Hérelle declined, citing, among other reasons, his health. At sixty-one, he suffered not only from persistent bronchitis but also from a variety of other ailments, some stemming from his travel in the tropics and others from his exposure to infectious agents. He had battled recurring bouts of malaria. Twice in his life he contracted amoebiasis, another form of dysentery, caused by amoebas. In Egypt, he developed a fever of unknown origin that plagued him for six months. His phrenic nerve, which controls the movement of the diaphragm and is essential to breathing, was damaged too. Bacteriophages weren't the only creatures he injected himself with. At some point, he had self-administered a shot of the tetanus bacteria, which caused the phrenic nerve paralyses.[41] With that assemblage of maladies, it's not surprising that he preferred the milder, subtropical Tiflis weather to Moscow's bitter, snowy winters and chilly, wet springs. Notably, however, neither weather nor illness ever stopped d'Hérelle from pursuing his goals. Perhaps above all, he preferred to work in the company of his Georgian colleague. He was looking forward to building the institute with his friend. The work-around for Beria's funding denial was in progress.

In 1935, still in Tiflis, d'Hérelle penned his last book, *The Bacteriophage and the Phenomenon of Recovery*. In this 273-page monograph, which he hoped would serve as a manual for Soviet medics and lab technicians, he summarized his lifelong work on bacteriophages and their clinical applications as living medicines.

In went the recipes for making proper meat bouillons. In went the directions for training bacteriophages on specific strains. In went the "contagious recovery" phenomenon. So did various studies d'Hérelle and Eliava performed together to elucidate phages' living nature and modus operandi. But more importantly, d'Hérelle outlined the phage treatment directions for the most common diseases of the time—a detailed and clear manual any physician could use.

By that time, d'Hérelle had used phages for a great variety of afflictions. In the book, he described ways of treating urinary tract infections by injecting bacteriophage solutions directly into the bladder. He cited good clinical results from using phages for gallbladder inflammations. He dedicated a section to *Staphylococcus aureus*, which Russian scientists dubbed the "golden staph" because it oozed out a yellow-orange pigment, staphyloxanthin. An often-commensal organism dwelling on people's skin, *S. aureus* could turn vicious, causing painful boils, called *furuncles*, or clusters of them, called *carbuncles*. At a time when many people still didn't have running water and daily showers were an unimaginable luxury, these infections were extremely common and sometimes formed entire colonies on the skin. Besides pain, the boils could become very dangerous when they ruptured, letting the golden staph escape into the bloodstream, which could lead to sepsis and death. Doctors usually cut the boils, squeezed out the pus, and sterilized the site with antiseptics. D'Hérelle suggested injecting the staphylococcus phage into them instead—like he did years ago with buboes—citing many successes by his colleagues and himself.[42]

He also discussed intravenous injections of phages for treating staphylococcus-triggered sepsis but noted that this method had short-lived yet drastic side effects. Patients usually reacted to phage transfusions with spiking fevers, violent shivers, and later with drenching sweats. About two hours later, their temperatures would drop, and they would start feeling better, with about 80 percent of them recovering, which was very impressive by the standards of the time. To decrease the shock symptoms, especially for patients in a very weak state, d'Hérelle suggested starting with very small transfusion doses and gradually increasing them. He even described two cases of curing children from staphylococcus meningitis—a disease that was 100 percent fatal at the time—by cerebrospinal phage transfusions.[43]

Cleverly, he made a point of touting the treatment benefits for the Red Army in a form of polyvalent bacteriophages—a cocktail active against staph, streptococcus, E. coli, and a few others. Wounds, he wrote, often got infected by multiple types of bacteria, so a mixture worked best. D'Hérelle called it a *pyo-phage* and noted that the surgeon Alexander Tsulukidze had already put some to use. He cited cases of a near-miraculous healing of shoulder and hip gunshot wounds, which included broken bones. Typically, such injuries festered for a long time, sparking high fevers and, if the infection spread, ending in death. In one case, the patient had gone through six surgeries in six weeks, looking worse every day. With phage applications to his inflamed tissues, the infection vanished within three days, as did the fever—and he recovered. "Pyophages are invaluable for treating war injuries not only because they heal fast and easy, but also because they don't require dressing the wounds very often," d'Hérelle wrote in the book. Once phages were in, they did the job themselves, killing the existing germs and guarding against any new invaders sneaking in from the dressing cloth. With pyo-phages, military hospitals would lose fewer soldiers and put them back on their feet faster, d'Hérelle noted. "All of these considerations make bacteriophages' application and prophylaxis extremely useful for frontline conditions."[44]

The moment the bacteriophage bible was done, Eliava was hard at work translating it from French to Russian and Georgian. Translating and typing over two hundred pages likely took weeks if not months. As he was working late hours, Amelia reproached him again. "Why are you always putting your efforts into other people's work?" she questioned. "Why are you translating his book? Why aren't you writing your own?" She felt that Gogi was missing his chance to make his own mark in science. He too could stage hundreds of experiments. He too could write down the results. He too could send the papers to prestigious journals. But he was always too torn and driven in multiple directions. "When will you focus on your own research?" she pressed.

"Just wait," Gogi placated her. "Just let me get over all this."[45] His days were consumed by fighting for barley and oats and bricks and an extra car. But now he felt he was getting close. With d'Hérelle's book, he was all but convinced that the dream was within his reach. Perhaps another couple of years. Perhaps three. And then he would have everything in one place—a hospital, a research facility, an epidemiological station, serving the people of his nation and anyone else who needed help. Then he could finally take a break, do his own experiments, and write his own book. For now, he had to focus on d'Hérelle's. It played a crucial role in his plan.

In the beginning of the book, d'Hérelle—whether by his own decision or likely in agreement with his friend—penned a strategic political preface. "I have written this book for the scientists of the USSR, the amazing country, which for the first time in the history of humankind choose to be led not by the irrational mysticism but a solid science outside of which there is no logic and there can't be true progress." His diplomatic overture didn't end there. D'Hérelle struck an even greater, stronger accord, devoting his lifelong work to the USSR's supreme leader. "I dedicate this book to the person who, driven by the unprejudiced logic of history is building a new human society based on new principles and has reached such obvious levels of success that an impartial observer has no doubt in his final result. I dedicate it to Comrade STALIN."[46]

Having finished his work, d'Hérelle once again headed to France in the fall of 1935 to check on his own lab. He had every intention to return the next year to continue their joint efforts. Irakli Georgadze, who bid the French couple farewell in Batumi, remembered that moment for the rest of his life. "A snow-white Italian ship called *Delmatzio*. A snow-white uniform on the captain." And d'Hérelle shaking his hand goodbye. "I am going to come back next fall," he said. "And you, Irakli, are going to be speaking French fluently by then, OK? Because I want you to go and work at the Pasteur Institute for a year or two. A real microbiologist should go through this school."[47]

The Bacteriophage and the Phenomenon of Recovery was published the same year, 1935, by the Tiflis University, sanctioned by its dean Levan Aghniashvili, the brother of Petre Aghniashvili, Eliava's former benefactor. And then Eliava played his winning hand of cards.

He asked Budu Mdivani—the friend he had grown close with in Paris and the former Red Army commissar—to take the book and the updated institute proposal to Moscow. There, Mdivani passed them to Stalin's right hand and another powerful Georgian, Sergo Ordzhonikidze, who in turn presented it to Stalin. There are no records that tell whether the book and the proposal arrived in Moscow at the same time. In fact, the proposal might have landed there first, shortly after Beria's refusal, and the book was the impetus for Stalin to respond. Or it might have been that the book was presented first and the proposal came second—a brick-and-mortar promise of the manuscript's ideas. Regardless of the order, both artifacts completely bypassed Beria. It was a courageous political game. And it worked. Spectacularly.

Not only did Stalin approve the budget, but he went above and beyond what Eliava asked for. The supreme leader designated not one, not two, and not even three million to the bacteriophage heaven but a true fortune. On April 14, 1936, SovNarKom committed 13 million rubles to the creation of an All-Union Bacteriophage Institute, along with a satellite complex. According to the 1936 exchange rate, that would amount to $2.5 million USD. Today, it would exceed the purchasing power of $50 million USD.[48] To that decree, Stalin added a slap in the face addressed to Beria. "Please provide all possible assistance."[49]

Eliava wasted no time. A team of designers including a well-known architect invited from Leningrad, drew blueprints for the institute buildings, bound into a massive, heavy volume that took two people to carry. From façades to the interior sections, each building was drawn in miniscule detail with impressive clarity and quality. Although the colors may have faded slightly, the colossal soon-to-be-century-old album resides in the Eliava Institute's archives today.

The campus design encompassed everything Eliava ever

dreamed of: a research facility, a manufacturing plant, an epide-miological station, and, of course, a world-class clinic. One of the largest buildings was a spacious, three-storied hospital that would fit four hundred to five hundred patients with only two per room—a comfort level rivaling modern Western settings. The blueprints also included apartment buildings for the institute staff and a special two-family residence for Eliava and d'Hérelle. Designed as a classic French cottage with sloping roofs, tall glass doors, and wooden window shutters, it would look like a charm-ing provincial home, hugged by wisteria and roses that grew so lushly in Georgia's subtropical climate. The institute grounds were already a marvel—Eliava had employed a renowned landscape ar-chitect, Mikhail Mamulashvili, who had studied his craft in France. With two separate entrances and six rooms each, the two collabo-rators would have an ample space to work on their reports or have dinners together. D'Hérelle would no longer have to stay in a hotel, and Eliava would have plenty of time to write his own scientific works.

In December 1936, after Tiflis was officially renamed as Tbilisi, the USSR People's Commissariat of Health approved all of the building plans. Construction began immediately. D'Hérelle, who had been injured in a train accident and was recuperating in the Riviera, didn't come that year as he originally promised. He did, however, send more equipment to the Bacteriophage Institute, planning to return soon. By then, the French cottage would be finished. In January 1937, the workers would start laying its foun-dation.

The dream was finally coming true.

6

The Great Terror

No, he is not here," Ganna said into the phone once again to the same man who had already called a few times asking for Giorgi Eliava. "He isn't back yet." The man would hang up—and call again shortly after, not once bothering to introduce himself. It should have been an ominous sign, but at the time, Ganna didn't think much of it.

An abundance of phone calls directed to Gogi was not unusual. He knew so many people and was involved in so many things, personal and professional, that the phone rang all the time. But in retrospect, the same man's persistent calls and his refusal to identify himself should have been alarming. Still, Ganna, a twenty-two-year-old senior student at the Geology Faculty of Tbilisi University, was too preoccupied with her own plans for the day. And they were quite important.

In the evening, Ganna's fiancé, Geno, would come to officially announce to her parents his intention to marry her. The young couple was anxious because Ganna's parents were somewhat disappointed in her choice—they thought their bright and beautiful daughter could have done better. To prepare for the evening, the couple had met at a mutual friend's house, and now Ganna was back home, waiting for her parents to return. It was 3:00 p.m., and they weren't back yet. The phone rang again. The same unfamiliar voice, the same familiar question.

The fateful day was January 22, 1937, Lenin's Memorial (he had died on January 21, 1924), and therefore, a holiday. Earlier in the day, Gogi and Amelia had taken a horse carriage to Saburtalo—a countryside journey to Tbilisi's outskirts. They wanted to watch the construction workers lay down the foundation for the French cottage, the future residence of the Eliavas and d'Hérelles. Leaving for the day, they were both filled with excitement, especially Gogi, who was imagining living minutes away from the labs, the hospital, and his friend. He would no longer have to spend his time running between four different locations or procuring bricks and oats. With Stalin's fortunes, the institute would soon develop an international reputation, and renowned scientists would flock there for conferences and congresses.

The Eliavas came back tired and hungry but delighted. With them came a guest, whom Ganna described as a new character who was constantly "hanging around Gogi"—in retrospect, likely a secret police goon. The dinner was waiting—the babushka served the appetizer of steaming boiled potatoes and herring, a classic Russian dish. At the start of the meal, the doorbell rang, but it wasn't Geno.[1]

In walked four people, some in civilian clothes, others in military uniform carrying with them the unmistakable aura of NKVD. Gogi impulsively jumped to his feet, but before he could utter a word, one of the four ordered everyone to remain seated. "Stay where you are." The men checked the "guest's" papers and dismissed him, quickly starting the search—*obisk*. Two of them disappeared into the bedroom with Amelia, combing through clothes and personal items. The other pair took over the dining room and the study, painstakingly leafing through books and magazines, searching for the *compromat*—compromising materials. After plowing through the classics and the encyclopedias, they dug into Eliava's desk, shuffling around his research papers.

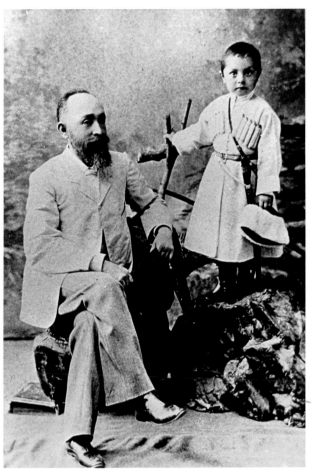

Giorgi Eliava, as a child in traditional Georgian clothes, with his father.

(Family archives of Natalia Devdariani-Malieva)

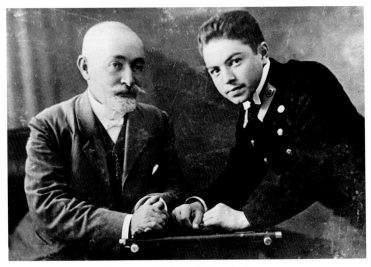

Giorgi Eliava at 15, with his father, after graduating from the gymnasium.
(Family archives of Natalia Devdariani-Malieva)

Giorgi Eliava, as a young man, with his father and sisters.

(Family archives of Natalia Devdariani-Malieva)

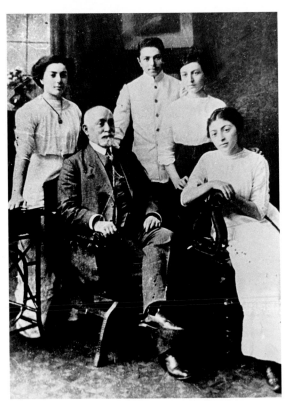

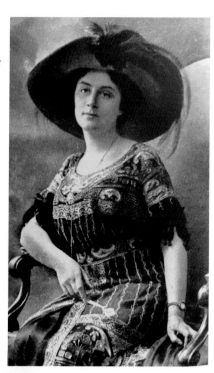

Amelia Wohl-Lewicka.

(Family archives of Natalia Devdariani-Malieva)

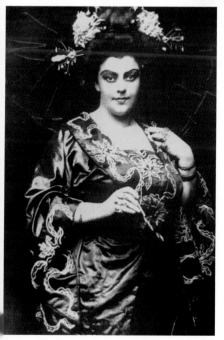

Amelia Wohl-Lewicka
on stage, circa 1910.

(Family archives of Natalia Devdariani-Malieva)

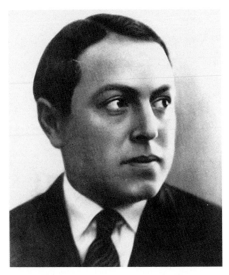

Giorgi Eliava, circa 1930s.
(Family archives of Natalia Devdariani-Malieva)

Félix d'Hérelle, circa 1905.
*(Service photo Institut
Pasteur—Photothèque)*

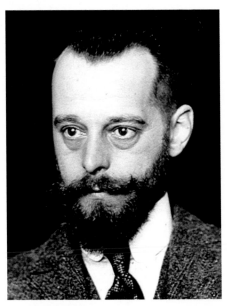

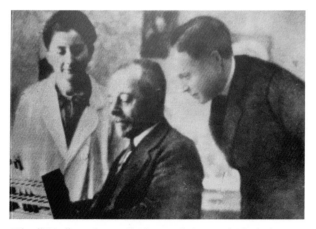

Félix d'Hérelle working with Eliava and Elena Makashvili, circa 1930s.

(Archives of George Eliava Institute of Bacteriophages, Microbiology and Virology)

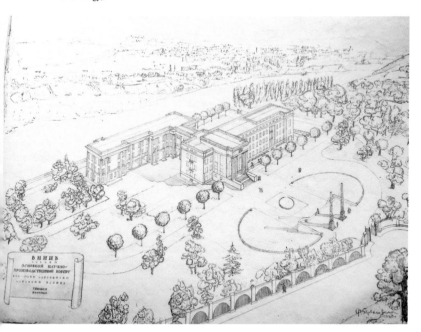

The Bacteriophage Institute plans, drawn in 1936 as part of Eliava's ambitious goals. The label states: The Main Science and Manufacturing Building.

(Archives of George Eliava Institute of Bacteriophages, Microbiology and Virology)

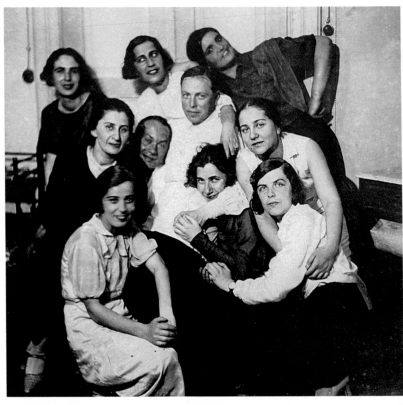

The last photograph of Giorgi Eliava, taken with his team a few days before his arrest.

(Archives of George Eliava Institute of Bacteriophages, Microbiology and Virology)

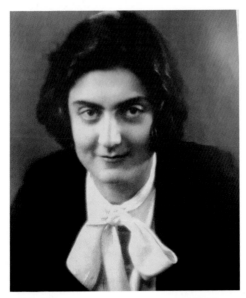

Ganna Eliava, as a young woman in 1936, before her arrest.

(Family archives of Natalia Devdariani-Malieva)

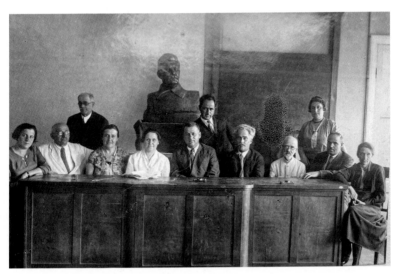

The dark, scratched-out part of the photograph had once been a person, possibly Giorgi Eliava, whose legacy had been meticulously erased from public records and public memories.

(Archives of George Eliava Institute of Bacteriophages, Microbiology and Virology)

Eliava's name crossed out on the title page of the architectural volume where he was listed as the director of the Bacteriophage Institute. Years later, someone stubbornly wrote his name back—in script.

(Archives of George Eliava Institute of Bacteriophages, Microbiology and Virology)

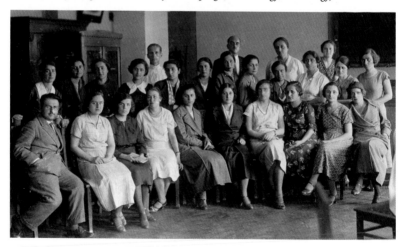

The institute team in 1938. Eliava employment views were gender-agnostic, and he often hired sisters, daughters, and wives of the persecuted, so they could feed their families. That practice laid the foundation for the organization's future. In the years that followed, female employees, students, and doctoral candidates often outnumbered male ones.

(Archives of George Eliava Institute of Bacteriophages, Microbiology and Virology)

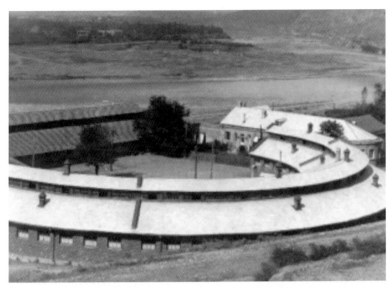

The first building of the Bacteriophage Institute built in Saburtalo (outside view).
(Archives of George Eliava Institute of Bacteriophages, Microbiology and Virology)

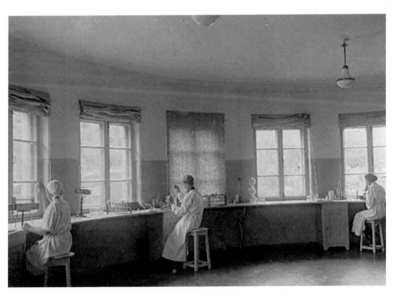

The first building of the Bacteriophage Institute (inside view). Women working in the vaccine department.
(Archives of George Eliava Institute of Bacteriophages, Microbiology and Virology)

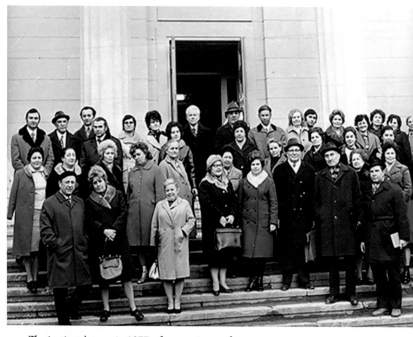

The institute's team in 1977, after a major conference.

(Archives of George Eliava Institute of Bacteriophages, Microbiology and Virology)

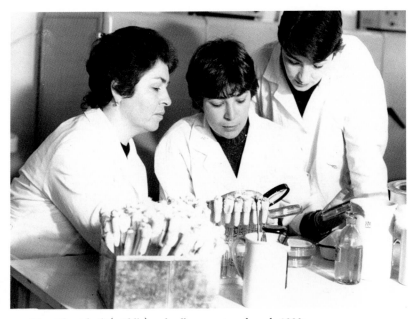

Nina Chanishvili (middle) and colleagues at work, early 1980s.

(Archives of George Eliava Institute of Bacteriophages, Microbiology and Virology)

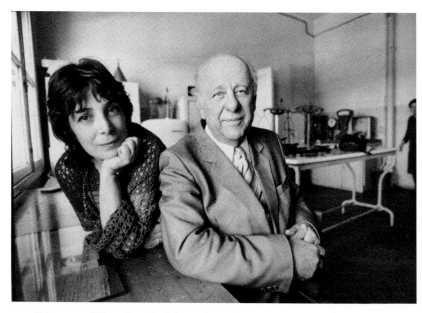

Teimuraz and Nina Chanishvili in 1996.

(Archives of George Eliava Institute of Bacteriophages, Microbiology and Virology)

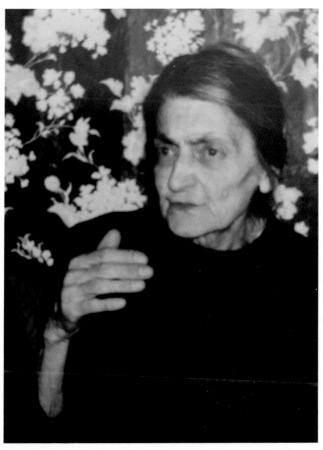

The last photo of Ganna Eliava, taken in 1997.

(Family archives of Natalia Devdariani-Malieva)

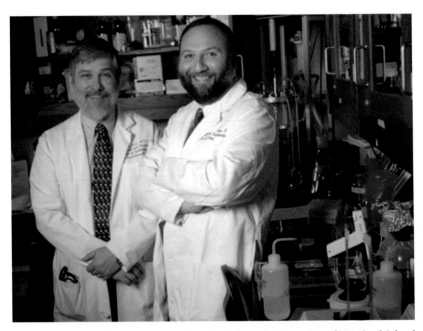

Glenn Morris and Alexander "Sandro" Sulakvelidze at the University of Maryland School of Medicine in Baltimore, circa late 1990s.

(Family archives of Sandro Sulakvelidze)

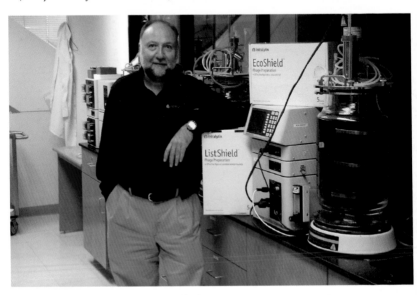

Sandro Sulakvelidze at Intralytix with phage sprays.

(Family archives of Sandro Sulakvelidze)

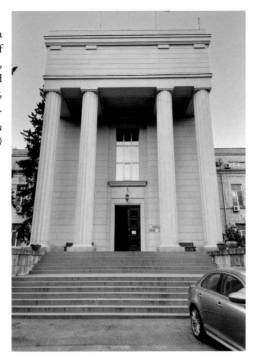

George Eliava Institute of Bacteriophages, Microbiology and Virology today, April 2022.

(Photo by Lina Zeldovich)

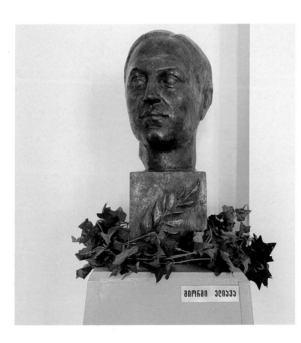

Giorgi Eliava's memorial inside the institute, April 2022.

(Photo by Lina Zeldovich)

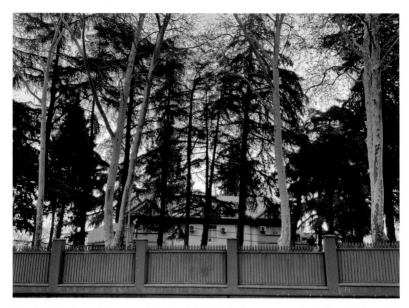

The French cottage, as it appears in April 2022, which was originally built to facilitate the collaboration of the two great minds, is still shrouded in mystery, hidden behind a tall fence. No one seems to know who owns it or what's inside.

(Photo by Lina Zeldovich)

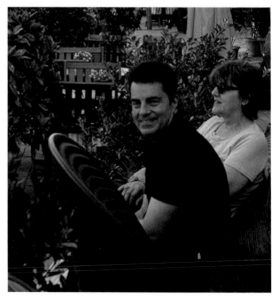

Natalia Devdariani-Malieva with son, Dimitry.

(Family archives of Natalia Devdariani-Malieva)

Gogi grew red in the face. Among the papers was a long, detailed presentation painstakingly prepared for an upcoming microbiology conference in Moscow, the symposium's centerpiece. "Please don't misplace my conference report," Gogi spoke, breathless and agitated. "I have to take it with me tomorrow." The officers showed no reaction, no acknowledgment. They already knew Eliava wasn't going anywhere. He didn't have a tomorrow.

The scene was so unreal that Ganna was struck by a strange thought. The search had to be fake! The men weren't NKVD officers but a group of cunning impostors—burglars and robbers, pretending to be the state officials to steal what they could. But they didn't seem interested in valuables. They were preoccupied with a different goal.[2]

The two-hour *obisk* revealed no *compromat*, but that didn't matter. The NKVD was accustomed to not finding anything worthy of arrest, but they took people away, regardless. After the 1934 assassination of Sergei Kirov, a party leader in Leningrad, the Soviet authorities passed a law that made searches, arrests, interrogations, convictions, and un-appealable death penalty verdicts much easier to implement. It became even more straightforward in 1937, so the goons needed no warrants, no legal authorizations, not even material evidence to whisk people away.[3] "You are coming with us," they informed Eliava while his horrified family watched helplessly.

He took it well, still confident and self-assured. "It's a misunderstanding," he told his family in his typical brisk style before he headed out into the hallway. "I'll be back soon." And then it must have finally sunk in, because he asked for another chance to say goodbye. Perhaps deep down he knew. Perhaps he read his fate on the men's faces. Gogi returned to the dining room and hugged his daughter and his wife. "Please take care of your mother," he said to Ganna. In his gut, he must have realized that this was not a misunderstanding. Not a mistake. In the past two months, others had been arrested too. Widely connected within the Tbilisi intelligentsia, he knew it better than anyone else.[4]

Thinking back, Ganna realized that the signs had been there all along. A month earlier, just as the building plans had been approved and construction began, several of Eliava's close friends were arrested, among them Vladimir Jikia and Budu Mdivani, who so graciously had delivered the proposal to the Kremlin. Eliava's patrons Petre and Levan Aghniashvili had been recently snatched also. In December, both of Ganna's parents were in Moscow—one on microbiology business and the other negotiating a performance contract—but then Gogi came back unexpectedly early and alone. When Amelia returned a couple of days later, the pair locked themselves in the bedroom and talked all night.[5] Were they talking about the arrests? Was Gogi worried he might be next? Or did he think that Stalin's patronage was a guarantee of his safety?

Ganna never knew the answer, but in retrospect, there was definitely something on his mind, something eating at the typically vibrant and endlessly optimistic Gogi. At an office birthday party that took place shortly before his arrest, he was uncharacteristically aloof, his usual bright smile gone, his typical exuberance extinguished.[6] In a picture taken that day, Gogi looks like a shadow of himself. He already might have known that the NKVD was after him. A free-spirited nonconformist, he stood out of the crowd too much—in more ways than one.

When the first wave of arrests swept up some of Gogi's friends, he was left furious and restless. "When it started happening, he was writing letters and petitions, asking to reconsider their cases," says Natalia Devdariani-Malieva. "He knocked on doors, he made phone calls, and he used every bit of his connections and power to help." People warned him to beware because "siding with the enemies of the people" would hurt him. "Don't stick your nose into that business," said the well-meaning folk. "Let it go. You will get yourself in trouble too."[7]

He didn't listen. He couldn't let it go. Not Gogi, who always fought for what was fair and right. So he did what he could. If he couldn't help those who had been arrested, he helped the families they left behind. "They were the people whom Gogi hired to work in the lab," Devdariani-Malieva shares. "The sisters, the daughters, the wives, so they could feed their children." Hiring relatives of the enemy of the people could backfire, but he didn't care. "Sometimes people came up to him on the street and told him, 'My husband was arrested, and we have no food left,'" says Devdariani-Malieva, "and he would reach into his pocket, pull a bunch of money, and give it out, without even counting."[8]

Now they came for him too. But in Eliava's case, they didn't stop there.

The door hadn't fully closed behind Gogi when the remaining two investigators took the women into different rooms. After a while, they called Ganna. "Stay with your mother for a few minutes." Limp and listless, Amelia was slumped in a chair, her huge hazel eyes staring into space. "Mama, stay strong, don't let yourself fall apart," Ganna began to say. Still looking into the distance, her mother took the golden watch off her hand and gave it to her daughter. "They are arresting me too."

Ganna grasped the watch in disbelief. "This can't be," she whispered. Her father's arrest was already devastating, but he, at least, was a public figure, always working with a myriad of people. Someone could've tipped the NKVD about some perceived wrongdoing, triggering the investigation. But arresting Amelia—the lyric-dramatic soprano who, outside of occasional performances, was a homebody, battling periodic bouts of polycythemia and the side effects of its medications—made no sense. Young and still idealistic about the Soviet system, Ganna looked for logic where there was none.

She hugged her mother goodbye in the hallway. "Don't worry, everything will be OK," she whispered. "That's what I should be telling you," Amelia answered—and then added quickly, "Go ahead, marry Geno." As she walked out flanked by the goons, Ganna's last look at her mother seared into her memory. "She was 52, but looked barely over 40, still stunning." She wouldn't stay that way much longer.[9]

THE ABYSMAL SPY NOVEL

"They came for me on April 3," Ganna wrote in her memoir decades later. They came late at night, pulling her out of bed and taking her away from Geno, whom she had married by then—a courageous act on his part when many people stopped talking to, calling, or even saying hello to Ganna, afraid to be associated with an enemy of the people. She was a month short of twenty-three, weeks away from earning her university diploma—and pregnant. "Consider moving back with your parents," the NKVD told Geno as they escorted his wife out to the NKVD building around the corner.

From January to April, Ganna had spent her time standing in long lines at the NKVD dungeon, trying to learn about the plight of her parents. The laws allowed relatives to bring clean clothes to the arrested and list the items on a piece of paper. The laws also allowed the jailed to send the paper back with their signature, acknowledging receipt. For those outside the jail walls, this small token of communication meant that their trapped relatives were still alive. For the imprisoned, it meant that their caring kinfolk was still free.[10] The accusations were typically a mystery, sometimes even for the investigators, who followed directives to take people into custody. One of the documents in Eliava's case reads "the material evidence for his arrest is not apparent."[11] None of it mattered. As a Stalin-era aphorism purported, "If there's a person, there's a statute." And therefore, a charge. And if there wasn't one yet, it was made up on the fly.

Sometimes family members learned that their relatives were shot by a firing squad after reading it in a newspaper, without a mention of where they were buried. Sometimes they deemed their kinfolk dead, but the missing would come back from hard labor camps a decade later, broken, but alive. And sometimes, people waited for their loved ones for years, refusing to give up hope, and never learned what really happened to them. During Stalin's purges, once you were "inside," there was no way out. The arrested had no rights to a lawyer or a fair trial. Acquittals not only were unheard of—they didn't exist.

In jail, Ganna made friends with prisoners of all ages, professions, and walks of life. A breastfeeding mother, forced to leave her newborn twins at home with a sickly grandmother, not knowing whether they would survive. A ninety-one-year-old woman who, when she was given a ten-year sentence to prison camps, told the judge, "Thank you for allowing me to live another decade." A high school girl whose entire class was arrested—and every boy was *prigovoren k rasstrelu*—sentenced to death by a firing squad. The prison cells were massively overcrowded—sometimes exceeding three people to a cot, and many slept on the floor or didn't sleep at all, with their health deteriorating quickly.[12]

One day, sick with fever in the jail hospital, Ganna spotted Tinatin Jikia, the wife of Eliava's best friend. Rightly or wrongly, she blamed the woman for her father's arrest, thinking that Lavrenti Beria must have viewed Gogi as a successful rival.[13] The reality was, of course, far more complicated. Beria was clearing up his own path to power, eliminating anyone who stood in the way, while also proving his allegiance to the supreme leader by eliminating spies and enemies of the people. Eliava fit the bill perfectly.

Did he travel abroad? Yes, to Paris, Berlin, and other places. Did he live in another country long enough to be recruited by its intelligence service as a spy? But of course, he lived in France, for years at a time. Did he commonly interact with foreign nationals? By all means—he was married to a Polish opera singer and regularly entertained a French couple, who could've been masquerading as Soviet supporters in their attempt to sniff out the readiness of the Red Army—or worse, poison it with toxic bacteria.

Ganna's interrogations began shortly thereafter, but for the most part, she was lucky. Her main interrogator was her former schoolmate, a grade older than she—a young and decent man, too gentle for his profession. She escaped the beatings, floggings, nails, and needles so common in NKVD methods. (Her parents were not spared.) Her inquisitor simply ran through the script. The questions didn't make any sense to Ganna, and the conversations always sounded like a broken record of insanity.

"What anti-Soviet nationalist groups did your parents entertain at home?"

"They didn't."

"When was your father first recruited by foreign agencies to spy for them?"

"He wasn't."

"What other anti-Soviet activity did your parents engage in?"

"They didn't."

"What sabotage and wrecking actions was your father planning to carry out?"

"He wasn't.

"What anti-Soviet conversation between your parents were you privy to?"

"None."

Late night in May, by accident, the jail personnel brought Amelia into the same cell as Ganna. Barely recognizable, she had gone from an elegant lady to "a skin-wrapped skeleton" in only three months. Sick with worry about her loved ones, she couldn't eat. Mother and daughter spent the night together, trying to make sense of what happened to them and Gogi, until the jailers recognized their mistake in the morning. The two got another chance to see each other after Amelia almost died in the jail hospital from a kidney infection. "If I live, can you put me with my daughter?" she asked the doctor, a kind soul who tried to help every person he saw, for which he was later *prigovoren k rasstrelu* himself. No one expected her to live, but she did—and the doctor kept his promise. In the summer of 1937, mother and daughter spent two weeks together in the same cell—the last time they saw each other.[14]

Toward the end of the year and still in prison, Ganna gave birth to a son. The boy, born with a strange bump on his spine, didn't live long—another life smothered and likely undocumented by the Great Terror. After Ganna was finally given her sentence, she spent eight years in the hard labor camps, freezing in the winter, suffering under heat in the summer, and battling everything from infections to injuries to fleas. "Only my youth and my desire to live got me through," she wrote in her memoir. That—and her hope that her parents were still alive—because it was simply counterproductive to eliminate such bright and talented individuals. "She convinced herself that Gogi was kept locked up inside a secret lab, working for his country from inside some sort of a prison, because killing him was a waste of a talent that the country needed very much," Devdariani-Malieva says. "She was hoping for some logic to exist." But she was wrong.

When she was allowed to return to Tbilisi—where her husband, Geno, had since moved on and where most people were still afraid to talk to her—she couldn't find any traces of her family.

Only years later, weaving together bits and pieces of information that came from different people at different times, was she finally able to restore the picture of what happened to Gogi and Amelia. It was like trying to piece together a shattered hand-painted vase, where the brightly colored fragments of human memories had scattered far and wide, and no matter how many you found, the rest were still missing.

THE NKVD'S "SPY NOVEL"

As much as Beria was vindictive, his real goal was much bigger than punishing his critics. A gritty careerist, he was determined to climb to the top, so he went after the person who stood in between him and Moscow: Budu Mdivani. It wouldn't be a straightforward task, but Stalin's paranoia and purges made it possible. One only needed to extract enough evidence from broken and tortured people to make the case look plausible on paper. And so the NKVD wheels were set in motion, slowly picking up speed.

The first two and a half months after his arrest, Eliava wasn't even questioned. His first interrogation, or *dopros*, occurred on April 3, the same day the NKVD arrested his daughter. Did he refuse to accept the accusations, prompting the goons to snatch Ganna? If there was a connection between the two events, records don't reveal it. Eliava's *dopros* record from April 3 doesn't seem to exist, but the subsequent documentation that refers to it mentions that he "agreed to stop his denials and give an honest confession."[15] The NKVD had its own definition of "honest" because the records from later *doprosi* read like a poorly narrated spy novel where the author constantly shifted the plot, chasing a new target each time.

The April 6 *dopros* record states that Eliava was recruited by the French intelligence while in Paris in 1926 and later introduced his superiors to Mdivani, who wanted to overthrow the Soviet government and viewed France as a helpful and willing force. The May *dopros* swapped France for England, supposedly because Eliava "confused" some of the facts. Later in June, he revealed that he was apparently an active agent of both, and had enlisted a Georgian colonel to help infiltrate the Red Army, paying him 500–600 rubles per an intelligence report. Operating under the pseudonym Othello and code 68, the number of people he supposedly recruited into his intelligence circles reached sixty-five—a massive network of spies who gathered information on the Red Army locations, its supply system, its military fitness, and its psychological readiness for battle.[16] The alleged snitches had established meeting places, safe houses, and a system of transferring documents and money in and out of Tbilisi through various embassies in Moscow. Eliava also allegedly admitted to channeling money into the Georgian National Center, led by Mdivani, with far-reaching goals—including overthrowing the Soviet government.

Later, the plot hit new levels of absurdity with the addition of a terrorist scheme. According to the June records, Eliava and Mdivani tried poisoning Soviet citizens by slipping *Clostridium botulinum*—a harmful bacteria that can proliferate in canned food—into the jars in Tbilisi's canning factory. With Mdivani's blessing, Eliava gave two bacteria-laden vials to the factory official, Mikhail Okudjava. Later in June, the NKVD staged *ochnie stavki*—specialty interrogations in which two battered, exhausted, and agonized individuals were pitted against each other and forced to add more twists to incriminate themselves. After an *ochnaya stavka* with the institute's head of the stables and vaccine department, Eliava allegedly admitted to poisoning rural wells with typhus bacteria (in fact, his team had been treating the wells with bacteriophages to prevent infections). He also stated that he and Mdivani were ready to launch bacteriological warfare against the Red Army in the event of war. Shockingly enough, there was one thing he declined to do, according to yet another *dopros*. In 1935, when Mdivani asked him to "carry out a terrorist act on Beria using bacteriological microbes," he refused.[17]

The *doprosi* documents, written as summaries, don't appear signed, so it is impossible to tell whether Eliava indeed pleaded guilty or whether the NKVD interrogators typed up whatever fit their agenda on a given day. Timothy Blauvelt, an American historian and professor of Soviet and post-Soviet studies at Tbilisi's Ilia State University, dug up the documents from the declassified KGB archives and found that interrogators had argued with one another about what they wanted Eliava to say. One of them accused the other group of taking the scientist's confessions in the wrong direction and "slowing down the investigation [of Eliava] by constantly redoing and rewriting the interrogation protocols."[18] Equally telling are their descriptions of the bioterrorism acts. "Given the crudeness of the supposed terroristic plots they concocted, involving the use of bacteria to poison essential resources such as wells, it seems clear that they had very little detailed understanding of the scientific principles involved," Blauvelt says.

It's possible that Eliava confessed many sins that he never committed. The NKVD stopped at nothing to force people to talk. Piecing together the information about her father's fate—from people who might've known him in jail or heard from others who had shared cells with him—Ganna had learned horrifying details of his last days. "They did terrible things to him," said one woman. "Things you can only do to a man."[19] Another person added more chilling descriptions. "If you only knew how they tortured him," he said. "They broke his arms and legs so he could barely move. He couldn't walk no more, couldn't stand up. He lived in constant agony, engulfed in pain. At the end, he had lost his mind to that pain and gone insane."[20] His death penalty verdict, given to him

July 6, 1937,[21] was a liberation. On July 9, a firing squad brought the end to his suffering.

In a great irony of timing, Gogi was shot during the two weeks Amelia and Ganna cherished in the same prison cell, one barely alive and the other pregnant. On one of those days, in the bathroom, Amelia found a ripped piece of newspaper that listed several "enemies of the people" who had been shot for their anti-Soviet crimes. One of them had the last name of Eliava, but because the initials were torn off, and because there were several other Eliava families in Tbilisi, and because the names of the other "criminals" were completely unfamiliar, Ganna was vehement this wasn't her father. She was so certain that it was another Eliava that she all but convinced her mother too. "I kept telling her that it was absurd, that it couldn't possibly be Gogi," she wrote in her memoir. "I was wrong. The absurd had taken place."

Whether Eliava surrendered to the accusations or not, his testimony and confessions were attributed to him anyway—and used against dozens of other victims in Georgia from 1937 to 1938, in part because he knew so many people who were easy to label as anti-Soviets. The NKVD officials were under tremendous pressure to expand their traitors list to meet the target numbers of arrestees.[22] "When you look back you realize it was just statistics," says Devdariani-Malieva. "The NKVD had the numbers they had to hit so they just did it. There was no sense in it, no logic." The "target numbers" were mind-boggling. Out of about two million Georgian citizens, over twenty-nine thousand were persecuted, with about half executed and the other half sent into hard labor camps. Stalin's purges were worse than any plague or infectious disease.

At the end of the cleansing, Beria gave a triumphant speech denouncing the traitors of the motherland as enemies of the people while glorifying the tireless work of the NKVD that kept the Soviet

Union safe and secure. His plan worked. In 1938, he was rewarded with a promotion to Moscow to continue his work there. From 1938 and until Stalin's death in 1953, he was the head of the secret police, in charge of liquidating the enemies of the people and overseeing the labor camp network.

Even when the Great Terror of 1937 subsided, the fear and horror it sowed among the people continued well beyond Stalin's and Beria's deaths in the 1950s. Later, the Soviet vocabulary forged creative euphemisms to refer to the victims. Those sent to camps or killed were called "the repressed." When the victims' good names were restored, they were said to be "rehabilitated" as if those who died could be brought back to life.

Both of Ganna's parents were found innocent in the late 1950s, after Stalin and Beria were gone. There were no crimes; no conspiracies; no plans to poison wells, people, or Red Army soldiers. When the documents of their arrests—at least those that could be found—were declassified, Ganna learned their verdicts. Her father's read *prigovoren k rasstrelu*. Her mother's case had an empty space where the cause of death should have been. Whether she was shot or died in prison, Ganna would never know. Nor would she ever learn where they had been buried. Both were "rehabilitated due to the absence of crime."[23]

When d'Hérelle learned of Eliava's arrest, he pleaded with Moscow but was informed, falsely, that his friend had already been tried and shot. Disillusioned and undoubtedly heartbroken, d'Hérelle had never returned to Tbilisi. He likely feared for his own safety too. Eliava's death dealt a huge blow not only to Soviet science but globally. As a research and treatment establishment, the Bacteriophage Institute would have exerted a major presence in the international scientific arena, but its reach was cut short. "The exposure of Eliava as a counterrevolutionary and spy, and the alienation of d'Hérelle, meant that the institute, although eventually becoming operational, would never gain such a status," Blauvelt writes.

The French cottage was finished, but it never became the happy house of the two great minds. In a bitter irony of history, it became property of the NKVD and later the KGB. Today, it stands behind a tall fence, hiding among the evergreen trees on an adjacent, but separate territory, still shrouded in secrecy. No one knows who owns it or what hides inside. The century-long mystery lives on, as if in mournful memory of its creator and his tragic fate.

The Soviet regime wiped out any real memories "the enemies of the people" left behind. Their achievements were obliterated. Their accolades and titles were taken away. Their personal property was confiscated. Their written works, diaries, and letters were destroyed. When the NKVD was done with Eliava, there was almost nothing left of his two decades of work. While he didn't publish often in scientific journals, he composed numerous reports, lectures, and lesson materials. During the twenty years of being the top microbiology figure in Georgia, he had educated a generation of medics, bacteriologists, and lab assistants. He had frequently spoken at symposiums and public health events. He was interviewed and likely photographed by the media. His name and signature appeared on the institute's documents, financial statements, and SovNarKom memos. Beria's goons succeeded in erasing his name, legacy, and image from nearly everything and everywhere. They expunged Eliava from public memory.

The vestiges of their efforts remain visible in the scant materials that survived. Eliava's name was carefully painted over in red on an expansive collaborative work about treatments for venereal disease, dated March 16, 1934.[24] With a series of X marks, it was also crossed out on the title page of the architectural volume where he was listed as the Bacteriophage Institute director. Years later, someone stubbornly wrote his name back—in script, above the Xs. Notably, d'Hérelle's name and title as a general consultant remained intact. It's not clear whether d'Hérelle's book that Eliava translated was removed from circulation, but only a few copies survived in private collections, despite the great risk.

A historical photo album that depicts the institute's early days holds several retouched black-and-white pictures. Taken at official meetings, they display a group of decision-makers at work. Upon close inspection, one can see that an attendee who once was part of the picture is no longer there. Instead of the face and body, there is a strange blackish cloud, hovering in the middle of the shot like an apparition. In these century-old pictures, it can be easily mistaken for a defect or just the wear and tear of time. But with an even closer look, it's clear that "the cloud" had once been a person, either meticulously scratched off or eaten by acid or other chemicals. "We don't know if this is Eliava or someone else," Nina Chanishvili says, "but it's very plausible that it was him. As the institute's leader he would've been at these official meetings." As the enemy of the people, however, he lost his right to appear in historical photos.

And yet, despite all, his name and his legacy lived. Eliava's dreams survived even though he perished in the NKVD prison. They lived in the memories of those who knew him. They lived in clandestine conversations of the people he had trained, hired, and helped. They lived in his ideas, accomplishments, and goodwill that his followers preserved and built on. The money for the institute's construction was already allocated, so some of it went on to build the phage research and manufacturing building. And while the treatment center never materialized, the phage production began shortly after. The living medicines were acutely needed because more trouble lay ahead. The battered country hadn't had a chance to heal from the Great Terror when something no less horrifying arrived: the Great Patriotic War, more commonly known as World War II. The Soviet people—some beaten into submission and others wholeheartedly believing in the great Communist future—now had to defend their country from Nazi invasion. In that international armed conflict, the costliest to date in terms of human fatalities, phages went on to save not only individual lives but major military missions.

7

Hell on Earth, Cholera in Water, Phages Underground

In the summer of 1942, a small plane was cautiously approaching Stalingrad when the pilots spotted a clear sign of trouble— German bombers quickly gaining speed. Stepping out of the cockpit, one of the pilots shouted to the six passengers sitting together on benches, "Can anyone operate a machine gun?" The only woman among them, slim with a short haircut, answered with a timid question. "What must we do—just spin the handle?"

The pilot gave her a look of contempt and turned around to head back to the cockpit. Just then, another passenger, a decorated general, cut in. "Are you out of your mind? Getting into a fight with these wings?" he shouted, implying that their plane couldn't maneuver well enough to fight the agile bombers. In a battle, it didn't stand a chance. "Hit the gas!" the general roared, certain it was the only way to shake the bombers off their tail. "Pick up speed!"

The pilot disappeared, and seconds later, the plane accelerated rapidly. It dove down fast, flying low, right above the Volga River's blue currents. The passengers fell off the benches, grabbing at whatever they could. But the maneuver did the trick—the bombers had lost their target. Shortly after, the plane landed safely on Stalingrad's airfield. The local head of NarKomZdrav's anti-epidemic department and a military epidemiologist waited on the tarmac to pick up the woman with the short haircut. And a bagful of phages.

The woman was Zinaida Vissarionovna Ermolyeva, a Russian microbiologist and bacterial chemist known for her work on infectious disease and phage medicines. Forty-four at the time, she managed to evade Stalin's purges of 1937 and was a leading researcher in the All-Union Institute of Experimental Medicine in Moscow, where she worked on discovering and making new therapies. Now, in the summer of 1942, when the German forces were closing in on Stalingrad—the Soviet stronghold on the Volga River—Moscow NarKomZdrav director Georgiy Miterev sent her here with an important mission to fight off a force more devastating than the Nazi troops closing in on the city: cholera.

At two o'clock in the morning, the team met in a small, stuffy room. The front line was only miles away, and the continuous cannonade racket reverberated through the closed windows. The explosions, loud, heavy, and close, shook the earth. Air raid sirens wailed. The bad news was that the front was approaching. The worse news was that cholera was most certainly approaching with it. The battlegrounds were still at a distance, but cholera was closer. Without a doubt, it was already floating in the Volga's currents.[1]

Earlier in 1942, the Soviet military command had learned about a cholera outbreak among the German Army. The news seemed good at first—the germ could devastate the enemy's battalions, bringing the Soviets their victory. But the euphoria was short-lived. Cholera didn't differentiate between the two fighting parties. It didn't respect front lines. It could cross over easily, hitching a ride in groundwater contaminated with infected feces, spilling into the river and sickening the entire city. If the epidemic engulfed Stalingrad, the Soviets would lose civilians, soldiers, and possibly the entire war. In 1942, Stalingrad was described by some as hell on earth. And in the midst of that hell, cholera was lurking in the water.

Stalingrad was a strategically important location for a myriad of reasons. A large city that stretched for about thirty miles along the west bank of the river,[2] it housed heavy industry. It was also a transportation and a military hub on a big bend of the Volga, through which thousands of people passed daily—from soldiers arriving to fight to civilians evacuating farther east to work in munitions factories. More importantly, the city sat right on the path to the oil fields of the Caucasus. The Caucasus's oil center of Baku—the same city where the absent-minded Eliavas nearly lost Ganna on their trip to Moscow—lay south from Stalingrad. By that point in the war, the Nazis were running out of fuel, and seizing Stalingrad would get them all the petrol they needed. The Soviets were equally desperate because the advancing Germans had cut off their other oil pipelines. If Stalin's army lost Stalingrad, stopping Hitler's march across the country would become immeasurably harder.

It was also a deeply symbolic battle site. Conquering the city bearing Stalin's name would signal victory to the worn-out German troops and defeat to the desperate Russian ones. But the opposite was also true—if Russians threw the Nazis off their vitally important city, the hopes for victory would soar while the Germans' morale would decline. The stakes were so high that to boost spirits, the führer had essentially told his nation that Stalin's stronghold was all but theirs—and with it the victory over Russia and Communism. And thus, the beautiful and atmospheric Volga city had become the focal point of the political and personal obsessions of two egocentric commanders. The battle over Stalingrad became a battle of ideas and beliefs. Whichever party seized the city would win the war.

The cholera threat raised the stakes even higher. In early summer of 1942, the city had a few confirmed cholera cases, indicating that it was only a matter of time before the epidemic blew up. The incessant air raids were steadily reducing the city to rubble. The few buildings that still stood were missing top floors. Ripped pipes stuck up from the crumbled pavement of the once wide, tree-lined streets. With the water mains destroyed and sewage systems shattered, both the drinking water supply and waste disposal systems were broken. People resorted to wells and latrines. With that, the old ghost of the nearly beaten deadly disease began to emerge. Stalingrad hospitals treated thousands of wounded fighters daily, and replacement troops arrived. Overcrowded steamboats and trains were continuously evacuating people to Astrakhan and Saratov, two nearby cities away from the front, and sometimes to other locales farther east. With so much traffic in all directions, the epidemic could freely trek to other parts of the country, hiding in travelers' intestines. It had to be stopped here, in its tracks, before it had a chance to wreak further havoc.

"Comrades," Ermolyeva said gravely as the team finished discussing the situation. "We must take immediate measures."[3]

When the sun rose, peeking through the heavy blue curtains, the team was still outlining the preventative measures. "We decided to give the entire population of the city and the troops stationed there a cholera bacteriophage," Ermolyeva recalled later. That amounted to thousands of people, but she did not have thousands of phage ampoules in her bag. She phoned to Moscow and asked her colleagues to ship as much bacteriophage as the institute could gather. The medicines were loaded up on the train, which left the capital shortly after, bringing the cure.

It never arrived.

On its final miles toward the city, the train was spotted by Nazi bombers that swarmed overhead, decimating it with their explosive wrath. There was little left of the munitions, provisions, or medicinal ampoules. Waiting for another train would take days, and there was no guarantee that it would make it. Ermolyeva's crew decided to organize the production of cholera bacteriophage right on the spot, essentially setting up a mini-factory. "It was not easy to establish a complex microbiological production in a besieged city," she wrote years later in her memoir, *The Unseen Army*. "It was necessary to produce the drug in huge, daily increasing quantities. We had to administer the phage not only to the local population, but also to thousands of people coming, leaving, and flying in and out of the city." The enormous responsibility, which could end up being the decisive force in winning or surrendering, kept her up late into the night. "It was hard to fall asleep right away, thinking about the immense task that confronted us, microbiologists, in the prevention of a terrible disease."[4]

Ermolyeva had high hopes for her colleagues at the Kharkiv Mechnikov Microbiology and Immunology Institute in Ukraine. It was the very team that once had agreed to collaborate with Eliava and d'Hérelle (or rather the surviving team, because its former leaders were arrested and shot according to the same Great Terror script). Previously located about five hundred miles west in Kharkiv, the institute had evacuated to Stalingrad months earlier and had the expertise to help with production. But with air raids and missile hits getting closer, the institute began to pack for another evacuation—the equipment and the scientists were too precious to risk being captured. Yet there was one thing Ermolyeva could count on: the phages themselves.[5] For as long as the Volga River was there, so were the tiny bacteria eaters, swimming in infinite supply. Ermolyeva's team didn't need special chemical reagents or complex machinery to synthesize the cure. They could grow it with basic lab equipment. So they set to work. In a basement of a destroyed building, they set up a makeshift laboratory and began to grow the living medicines underground. With the constant bombing, it was the safest place to raise them too.

As phages began to proliferate in their underground lab, Ermolyeva's team launched a massive awareness campaign, recruiting everyone who remained in the city. Volunteers and medical students went from house to house and apartment to apartment, explaining the dangers of cholera and the benefits of preventative "phaging." They kept a close watch on residents, checking for cholera symptoms and assuring that Stalingraders were phaging regularly. They tirelessly talked about the prevention of gastrointestinal diseases in ports and bomb shelters. They stood guard at stores where people came for food. They took watch at the evacuation centers, making sure that those leaving the city were properly phaged so that the disease couldn't travel with them. Everyone had to carry a phaging card. "It was impossible to leave the city without a certificate of phaging," Ermolyeva recalled. "Even the bakeries wouldn't give out bread without that paper."

To establish a successful prophylaxis, people would have to drink the cocktails on a fairly regular basis. That required uninterrupted phage production and continuous distribution. "Fifty thousand people took the bacteriophage daily," Ermolyeva wrote. "This has never happened before in history."

With radio and newspapers joining the awareness campaign, no one was left uninformed. One day, when Ermolyeva went down to the riverbanks to fetch some water for lab research, a little boy ran up to her. She had just dipped her bottle into the river when the child chastised her about being ignorant and careless. "*Tetya*," he called out to her with the Russian equivalent of "ma'am" used to politely address an older woman. "Can't you see, it's written everywhere here: 'Don't swim and don't drink un-boiled water!'"[6] She left the riverbanks happy. Even the children had learned the drill. Her lifelong quest to beat cholera was working in a war-torn Stalingrad.

Ermolyeva was born in 1898 to a family of Cossacks, a culturally unique group of people that made their home in the vast steppes surrounding the Black and Caspian Seas. Formidable and fiercely independent, the Cossacks were skilled horsemen and experienced warriors who successfully fought the Ottomans for decades. Even the czar had left them alone, except when recruiting them for military service, during which they plundered and pillaged like pirates. The youngest of six children, Ermolyeva grew up in a village of Frolovo, only one hundred miles from Stalingrad, which once was called Tsaritsyn. Her father, Vissarion Ermolyev, a military man like most Cossacks, died when she was twelve. Her mother—a woman well educated for her time who could read and write—sent her daughter to attend a gymnasium from which Ermolyeva graduated with high honors, a gold medal. In 1916, the same year Eliava was expelled from Odessa University, Ermolyeva was accepted into the medical school in Rostov-on-Don, another city in the Russian south. There, she fell in love with microbiology and had more ideas than she had time to pursue. "As a student, I used to climb through the laboratory's window in the wee hours of the morning before the building opened. Everything was closed, but I wanted to spend a couple of extra hours doing my experiments."[7]

According to lore, she chose cholera as her research subject because the scourge took the life of her favorite musical composer, Pyotr Ilyich Tchaikovsky. She had read his biography in school. At her gymnasium's graduation ball, the music band played Tchaikovsky's "Sentimental Waltz," and she decided to study medicine. In 1922, Rostov suffered an epidemic, originating from the polluted waters of the Don River and Temernik, its tributary. In one of the experiments, Ermolyeva isolated some cholera-like vibrions from the Rostov tap water and decided to test whether they would turn into the real *Vibrio cholerae* in human intestines. As many scientists did, she chose herself as the subject of this test. She drank the vibrions and promptly fell ill. She was lucky to recover and finish her experiment, writing down its findings: "An experiment that almost ended tragically proved that some cholera-like vibrions, while in the human intestine, can turn into true cholera vibrions that cause disease." At the end, she triumphed over cholera by writing recommendations for chlorine treatments of potable water.[8]

In Stalingrad, her team was winning the microbial war, but the success of the military one was still in question. Throughout the summer of 1942, the Germans kept advancing, closing in day by day and inch by inch. The city was forever shrouded in a veil of thick black smoke and the earth never stopped shaking from continuous explosions. The front line shifted, encroaching the city itself. Soon the battles would move onto the streets, and every building would turn into a battleground. "With pain, I watched the city being reduced to rubble, its beautiful buildings turned to ruins," she would write later.[9]

In late July 1942, the city was in full defense preparation, with about 180,000 civilians digging trenches, building fortifications, and barricading streets. Industrial equipment and livestock were being transported to the east side of the river, away from the front. At the end of August, Stalin decreed that the Soviet Army would hold the city at any cost, and he ordered a stop to the evacuation of industry in order to suppress any doubt in their victory. Historians would later write that with that decision, Stalin committed his nation to one of the most terrible battles in the history of war. The ferocity of the German attack was matched only by the tenacity of the defense.[10] Retreat was not an option.

The savagery of the battles and the brute force of the German troops was felt everywhere, and most acutely at the hospital where the wounded soldiers were treated and where Ermolyeva lived—in a small apartment near the operating room. In the beginning, surgeons removed bullets and stitched wounds there, but later, the incessant air raids destroyed the room—the bombs shattered the windows. Running out of space to house the wounded indoors, the staff turned the operating room into a ward, despite its broken windows. With more soldiers coming in, the hospital wards spilled into the backyard and garden. Ermolyeva could measure the mounting toll by the increasing number of cots that nurses had to fit into the same enclosures. The space between the cots was steadily decreasing.

Medics often treated soldiers' wounds with phages, in addition to common antiseptics. The method was widely tested even before the Nazi invasion, during the so-called Winter War between the Soviet Union and Finland in 1939 and 1940. As the conflict progressed, Professor Alexander Tsulukidze, who had worked with d'Hérelle and read his book in Eliava's translation, flew to Leningrad with an arsenal of phage remedies. With no lack of test subjects wounded by bullets, bombs, and mines, and complicated by severe infections, his team essentially ran clinical trials comparing phages to the "conventional therapy" of antiseptic solutions and salves. Just like d'Hérelle suggested, they sprayed phages on wounds and dressed them in phage-soaked gauzes. Sometimes they also gave soldiers phage shots. When treated with living medicines, wounds didn't need any follow-up; with the conventional therapy, however, doctors sometimes had to surgically remove more of the infected tissue. After three or four phage applications, the fevers dropped, and a week later, the wounds would start to close. With conventional therapy, that healing process took several weeks.[11]

A common scourge that settles in wounds is *Clostridium per-*

fringens, anaerobic bacteria that doesn't need oxygen to live. Unlike oxygen-loving aerobic germs that stay close to the wound surface and are easier to kill with topical antiseptics, *C. perfringens* squirms deep into the tissues where these remedies can't reach. Once it takes hold, its toxins kill flesh and release a rotten-smelling odor, which earned the disease its spine-chilling name: gas gangrene. Essentially eating the body from the inside, gas gangrene was very lethal in the pre-antibiotic era. When treated with phages, which penetrated the tissues following their bacterial food, the wounds healed significantly better and patients typically survived. The sooner their injuries were treated with phages, the faster they healed.[12]

Patients with broken bones relied on phages too. With conventional therapy, their casts were put on after their wounds were sterilized with antibacterial solutions like alcohol or iodine. But after a while, bacteria would settle underneath the cast, causing a foul smell. The casts had to be removed and the offensive gel-like pus had to be cleaned before a new cast was set. At the suggestion of one of the doctors who believed that phages would continue eating the germs underneath the cast, the crew began to spray bone injuries with living medicines. The idea worked—phages settled in, chewed up the bugs, and eliminated the need for repeated castings.[13]

Overall, Tsulukidze observed that phage therapy decreased the need for extra surgical interventions and thus the emergence of new infections. That spelled good news for both surgeons and soldiers who sometimes had to be transported from one hospital to another, extending their period of suffering. Instead, they recovered faster and were ready to go back to service sooner,[14] just as Eliava and d'Hérelle had once foretold. Eliava's name may have been expunged from documents and public memories, but the Institute of Microbiology, Epidemiology, and Bacteriophage that he started was growing phages that kept the army going. "The institute was a major supplier of phages to treat lacerations, gangrene, and intestinal infections at frontline hospitals," Chanishvili wrote in her recent paper "Professor Giorgi Eliava and the Eliava Institute of Bacteriophage."[15] Eliava's vision lived on.

Yet in war-ravaged Stalingrad, the phage injections Ermolyeva administered to soldiers were imperfect. Sent from Moscow, the phages produced inconsistent results. A few soldiers convalesced, but many still lay in feverish delirium, the sepsis-causing bacteria proliferating in their blood. It was likely because the phages in Ermolyeva's arsenal were active against certain bacterial strains and not others, but in the chaotic conditions of the besieged city, she didn't have the time to isolate the culprits and cultivate a more potent alternative. Just like d'Hérelle noted, it took time, skills, and precision—often impossible luxuries in the time of war.

No, that's not the remedy that can save people from sepsis caused by gun wounds, Ermolyeva thought. *We need something more powerful and more consistent.* She was thinking about her recent experiments with mold cultures that hindered bacterial growth. She had read about English scientists who isolated an antibacterial medicine called *penicillin* from the *Penicillium notatum* mold, a type of fungi,[16] but she didn't know where to find it. Together with her assistant Tamara Balezina, they went mold-hunting, trying out hundreds of species. One after the other, the multicolored fungi flourished in their petri dishes, but none seemed to kill bacteria, dampening the women's spirits.

One day, when the two were hiding in a damp bomb shelter from a German air raid pummeling Moscow, they noticed a bluish-green fungi growing in a crack of the wall—a new one they hadn't tried yet. After the explosions raining above their heads stopped, they carried the new specimen to the lab. When the bluish-green shelter species puffed up in the dish, it oozed a yellow substance as if surrounding itself with a protective ring that seemingly stymied the growth of various germs. It was indeed the *P. notatum* species

whose antibacterial properties Alexander Fleming first discovered in 1928 but didn't think of as medicinal.[17] "Would that kill
the germs inside a human body without side effects?" Ermolyeva
wondered while she stayed up late, thinking. She needed to get
back to her Moscow lab and resume the experiments.

"The nights were the worst," she wrote in her diaries. "Coming
home from work late evenings, I saw more changes happening in
the hospital and the anxiety's iron grip tightened around my heart.
Every night I woke up many times from noise, stomping and other
clamor. The window of my small room, located next to the operating room, overlooked the street leading to Beketovka, one of the
southern districts of the city. Outside, farmers rushed skinny exhausted cows and sheep to safer places. The sheep bleated mourn-
fully, as if calling out for help. I stood at the window for a long
time, then tried to lie down, only to wake up again."[18]

She had myriad thoughts on her mind. Besides the phage production, the approaching Germans, and the wounded soldiers moan-
ing in the garden ward, she was thinking of her two husbands—one
former, one current, both prominent microbiologists arrested by
the NKVD and rotting in jails. If they were still alive.

In 1925, Ermolyeva had been invited to Moscow to organize
and lead her own department at NarKomZdrav's Biochemistry
Institute. She packed only one suitcase, containing five hundred
cultures of cholera and cholera-like vibrions, and headed to the
capital.[19] She may have even crossed paths with Eliava, who was
on his way to Paris with family in tow. It would have been almost
inevitable for them to meet in the small world of Soviet microbiology, but because so many documents and diaries were destroyed,
there is no record of a meeting, if one occurred.

In Moscow, Ermolyeva met her future first husband: rising-star
virologist Lev Zilber. She married him two years later when they
both were on a long business trip in Europe. But their union was

short-lived. In 1930, Zilber left to head a microbiology institute in Azerbaijan, and their marriage fell apart. After a long period of heartache, she married prominent bacteriologist Alexey Zakharov, who had been in love with her for a long time. Both men were arrested during Stalin's purges with charges eerily familiar to Eliava's. One was allegedly conspiring to kill Soviet citizens by poisoning the water mains with encephalitis germs, and the other accused of sickening the horses to sabotage the production of serums.[20]

It is miraculous that Ermolyeva was never jailed herself. Some sources say that she was always ready for that moment. She kept a small suitcase, always packed with her most important items, in case the NKVD knocked on her door in the middle of the night. Rumor had it that Stalin simply *liked her* and even asked her for advice. He called her *sestrenka*—little sister.[21] Although not directly related—he hailed from Georgian mountains and she from Ukrainian steppes—Joseph Vissarionovich and Zinaida Vissarionovna serendipitously shared the same rare *otchestvo*, or middle name, inherited from their fathers. Stalin allegedly had the nerve to ask her which of her imprisoned husbands she would prefer to see free again. "Lev Zilber," she supposedly replied. Stalin was shocked. "But he is your ex. He's never coming back to you. He's married to another woman." Ermolyeva replied that "science needs him." Coincidence or not, Zilber was in fact set free, and more than once. Altogether, he was imprisoned three times, and Ermolyeva worked tirelessly to get him out every time. Zakharov died in prison, shortly after his arrest, but she didn't find out until after the war ended.[22]

Ermolyeva had become one of the country's leading authorities on infectious disease right before the war. Two years after Eliava's execution, the Tbilisi Institute of Microbiology, Epidemiology, and Bacteriophage officially opened, but because many of its buildings were still under construction, it couldn't yet meet its ambitious phage production goals. So Ermolyeva asked Nar-KomZdrav to let her expand phage operations in Moscow. She wrote a report explaining phage therapy successes and challenges. "She wanted to improve the overall quality of phage production, following d'Hérelle's criteria,"[23] says Dmitriy Myelnikov, a historian of science and medicine at the University of Manchester.

Studying phages' biochemical modus operandi was essential. So was upping production. Emphasizing that phages were crucially important for the health and security of the socialist state, Ermolyeva proposed to the NarKomZdrav to organize cholera phage manufacturing in both Moscow and Tbilisi, and to improve their quality. Her team had also experimented with various prophylactic measures, pouring phages into wells at the country's Afghan borders.

The prewar efforts to boost phage production had paid off in more places than Stalingrad. Soldiers going into battles carried phage vials in their kits, for wounds and intestinal disease. Civilians who managed to stash a few lifesaving ampoules held on to their treasures. In Leningrad, another besieged city that lasted through the nine hundred days of German blockade during which food was rationed to 125 grams a day,[24] phages saved people from the "hunger diarrhea" likely caused by dysentery from unsanitary conditions. Soviet author Boris Strugatsky, who penned many science fiction classics with his brother, Arkady, wrote his memories of the Leningrad blockade. "Then, in March, I came down with the so-called bloody diarrhea, an infectious disease that is dangerous even for a big grown man, and I was eight years old, and had dystrophy, which would be a certain death, one would think. But our neighbor (who also miraculously survived) somehow happened to have a vial of bacteriophage, so I lived."[25] Another blockade survivor, Irina Zelenskaya, who worked at the Seventh State Power Station, wrote in her postwar memoirs about visiting a colleague sick with colitis in the hospital. "I help him out a lot, to the extent that I got him some bacteriophage."

After Ermolyeva's efforts in Stalingrad stopped cholera in its tracks, NarKomZdrav wanted her to implement the same measures in other places. She became such an important figure in cholera prophylaxis that NarKomZdrav sent two planes to fetch her, but both were shot down. The third one, a little ambulance aircraft, made its way in by night. Ermolyeva rode to the airfield under the ongoing air raid and artillery shelling and was airborne in minutes. "Why are you staying so low?" she wrote a note to the pilot. "You'll get caught up in the trees."[26] "Better the trees than the bombers," the pilot wrote back. And he was right. The little air ambulance made it through by a sheer miracle. Fifteen minutes after takeoff, a crew of bombers descended from the sky and turned the airfield into a mass of churned dirt. Stalingrad battles would rage on for months, with thousands of casualties, but not from the dreaded intestinal scourge.

Barely touching down in Moscow, Ermolyeva was sent off to implement phage measures in another Volga city, Astrakhan. Now that she had a well-established procedure, the efforts went faster, and soon she was heading back to the capital. On the way, her airplane's motor overheated. The aircraft tumbled from the sky and crashed, breaking its wing. By another miracle, both pilots and Ermolyeva survived—only to fly to yet another war-torn city to fight cholera.[27] Full of promise, the bluish-green mold was burgeoning in her lab, but she was too busy to lay her hands on it. It was weeks before she was finally able to come back to her experiments.

When she did, *P. notatum* proved to be extremely successful. The yellowish substance it exuded was the very penicillin that destroyed bacteria faster and more consistently than anything else. Ermolyeva's team called it *krustozin*. After testing it on mice, guinea pigs, and horses, they reached out to clinical collaborators, who quickly tried krustozin in humans. "With great trepidations we waited for their first results," Ermolyeva wrote. And they were spectacular. The ooze seemed to kill just about any bacterial life. It stopped infections in burns, in wounds, and around broken bones. It even treated other, nonwar diseases like scarlet fever. And most importantly, it could be administered intravenously and through injections without the shocklike side effects associated with some of the phages. "Every Thursday physicians, surgeons, neurosurgeons, skin doctors and pediatricians gathered in my office to report their treatment results," Ermolyeva wrote—and they reported "bringing people back from the dead" with no exaggeration. "The range of penicillin antibacterial properties was incredibly impressive!" The news spread quickly, and Ermolyeva's lab started getting mailbags of letters from wounded soldiers begging for a vial of the wonder drug.[28]

Keeping up with demand, however, proved difficult. Remedies that work in petri dishes often don't work in big vats. Ermloyeva's crew organized a penicillin factory, but mass-producing was challenging. At about the same time, British scientists Howard Florey and Ernst Chain, in collaboration with the US Office of Scientific Research and Development, devised a factory production process for penicillin fermentation. In the winter of 1943, a small Anglo-American delegation of scientists that included Florey arrived in Moscow to establish contacts and work with Soviet physicians on medical topics and techniques, including the new wonder drug.[29] During that Moscow visit, the Soviet authorities presented the collaborative penicillin trials as a friendly competition between the two organizations. Florey called Ermolyeva "Madam Penicillin," but the parties disagreed which trial was most efficient. The Soviets struggled to mass-produce their krustozin, so eventually they bought a penicillin license from the Western scientists.[30]

Florey was skeptical about phages. "It is impossible to estimate what this phage work amounts to. Much of it, I feel, belongs to the 'Impressionist' school of science," he wrote.[31] The Soviets weren't ready to part with their phage secrets and their Western colleagues weren't going to accept it as a legitimate therapy until they knew the details.[32] What Western medics knew from their own literature didn't look promising.

By the mid-1940s, Western phage treatments were largely discredited. Some simply weren't a good match for the infections they were used to treat. Some made false claims promising to cure ailments that weren't caused by bacteria. And others might have been downright fake because there was not enough oversight from the regulatory bodies. Western medicine was a business, and because making potent phages took considerable time and work, the quality often suffered. The less scrupulous preparers may have done fewer passes than d'Hérelle would find acceptable, or perhaps they didn't bother to check the degree of their phages' activity against the target germs. There was no consistency in how polyvalent phages, which contained multiple phage types, were made—some were grown separately and mixed later, others were mixed in the beginning and grown together. Some concoctions had so much preservative in them that they deactivated the phages entirely.[33] The efficacy of phage medicines varied greatly.

Between 1934 and 1945, the *Journal of American Medical Association* published three reports, all of which deemed phage therapy highly unreliable. The most damning one was written in 1943 by Monroe D. Eaton and Stanhope Bayne-Jones, well-regarded figures in the medical world.[34] The two authors examined some of the existing bacteriophage literature and deemed it unsuitable for a standard of care therapy for several reasons. The preparations were capricious and often didn't work. When they did work, the scientists didn't have a control group, so it was impossible to know if it was in fact the bacteriophage that helped. Researchers commonly couldn't make phages work in mice or rabbits, which complicated testing protocols. A body, whether human or animal, interfered with bacteriophage ability to kill bacteria, so even when experiments worked in a dish, they failed in living creatures. Finally, the report noted that intravenous phage injections were dangerous and sometimes resulted in fatalities.

Notably, Eaton took over d'Hérelle's position at Yale University after the cantankerous scientist departed for Tiflis, says Ryland Young, professor emeritus at Texas A&M University, who spent over forty years studying basic phage biology. Eaton then went on to coauthor the report with Bayne-Jones, another medical mogul. "The report was effectively a hit piece on d'Hérelle," Young says. The report ended with a statement that could have been interpreted as a call for more research. "This is merely a reiteration of d'Hérelle's theory of the role of bacteriophage in immunity to infectious disease, a theory that at present lacks experimental support," the authors wrote. But in reality, it didn't usher any new phage investigations. Instead, it all but drove nails into the living medicines' coffin.

The pharmaceutical industry also played a role. Even those companies that manufactured phages in the 1920s and 1930s switched to antibiotics in the postwar era. Synthesizing molecules that consistently worked the same way was easier and cheaper than growing and training finicky creatures with picky appetites, whose biology scientists still didn't fully understand. Physicians agreed. At the time, a large percentage of American doctors were private practitioners. Many worked from their home offices and weren't attached to any bacteriological laboratories or hospitals.[35] They often didn't have adequate access to test labs, let alone complex facilities that could synthesize medicines as fussy as phages. In these settings, the easy, ready-to-use medications that had a long shelf life and killed a wide spectrum of germs were bound to win. Antibiotics offered all of the above. Reliable, repeatable, stable, and with no significant side effects known at the time, they phased phages out of use. Finally, Western doctors were suspicious of Soviet medicine. "Any science, good or bad, embraced by 'commies' was dangerous," Summers writes.[36]

On the contrary, in the Soviet Union, medicine was a state endeavor. A family couldn't start a company to grow phages or make penicillin. Medical school graduates couldn't open a private practice. Owning private business was illegal. Everyone was employed by the state, and all medicines were made at research institutions or large, state-owned factories. That made it harder to produce false advertisements, especially when the director's head was on the line. If their products didn't work or, worse, made patients sicker, they could be declared an enemy of the people. Stalin's regime imposed self-checks that were unimaginable in Europe or America.

Consequently, Soviet scientists followed a very different medical paradigm. Western medics embraced stability—in life, in laws, and in antibiotic drugs—but their Soviet colleagues learned to exist in an ever-shifting landscape. While penicillin was mass-produced today, it didn't preclude the factory from closing tomorrow. The raw ingredients could vanish. The inventor could be arrested. An institution could be shut down for espionage, wrecking—the Soviet term for destroying socialist property—or other crimes. Therefore, they used what worked and what they had on a given day.

Phages also fit nicely into the Soviet warrior ethos. The miniscule creatures were such mighty fighters that they destroyed bugs much larger than themselves. They sneaked in like scouts. They infiltrated the germs like spies. They destroyed from the inside. They were humanity's allies in the never-ending war against microbes. They had all the qualities of a good revolutionary and a country's patriotic defender. D'Hérelle's phage ideas also aligned well with the views of the revered Russian-Jewish Nobel laureate Ilya Metchnikoff, the grandfather of the microbiome theory, who posited that intestinal bacteria, such as acidophilus, play a huge role in human health.[37] He believed that by introducing enough good bacteria into the gut, one can not only fight off disease but even slow down aging—a century before scientists worldwide began to come to similar conclusions. For Soviet medics who wholeheartedly embraced his ideas, phages fit perfectly into that symbiotic view of humans and microbes. When in August 1960, two dogs, Belka and Strelka went up in space in the *Sputnik-2* spacecraft, they weren't the only ones inside this vessel. They were accompanied by an eclectic assemblage of "passengers," including mice, rats, fruit flies, bacteria, fungi, and two types of *E. coli* bacteriophages. Soviet scientists considered them important enough to see how they would fare through their cosmic journey.[38]

In the West, the last surviving commercial phage medicines disappeared by the 1970s. Ironically, by then, the first signs of antibiotic resistance began to appear. But in the Soviet pharmacopeia, phages held strong, saving lives when antibiotics failed.

8

The Rise of the Superbugs

In November 1956, doctors and nurses at the maternity ward of the Valley Hospital in Ridgewood, New Jersey, were worried.[1] An attractive modern facility designed to make the birthing process as easy as possible for mothers and infants, the hospital was battling a seemingly endless *Staphylococcus aureus* outbreak. The first signs of trouble appeared in 1955 when some mothers and babies developed skin infections. The nursery staff started washing their hands with hexachlorophene antibacterial soap and sterilizing linens in autoclaves. The incidence of infections dropped—only to increase a few months later, afflicting about 10 percent of infants and mothers. To make matters worse, the cases became much more severe, even life-threatening. By 1956, staph infections were causing pneumonia and breast abscesses.[2] And they didn't seem to respond to penicillin.

When two babies born at the Valley Hospital died of staphylococcal pneumonia in late 1956, the despairing staff started giving newborns a new antibiotic called *erythromycin* immediately after birth and for seven days. But some babies developed skin infections regardless. To the medics' horror, they soon found erythromycin-resistant staphylococci even in babies who weren't sick, confirming that the unkillable germ had taken a firm hold in the nursery.[3]

Similar outbreaks afflicted many hospitals across the United States at around the same time. In 1955, hospitals in Washington

State struggled with *S. aureus,* which plagued their patients with pustules, skin rashes, and breast abscesses.[4] One study found that out of 19,000 babies delivered in King County, 4,000 became severely ill, as did 1,300 women who gave birth. Jefferson Davis Hospital in Texas reported 16 newborn deaths, but a later investigation found that the outbreak was much larger—it infected 400 and killed 28 babies and 8 other children. In Manhattan, the New York Hospital was sending babies home only to readmit them shortly thereafter with abscesses and bone infections previously unheard of in infants.[5] From California to Iowa to Pennsylvania, hospitals were battling the new staph, and they weren't winning.

Exactly how this problematic strain arose wasn't clear, but it became a formidable threat, covering some with skin boils and killing others with pneumonia or sepsis. Initially, it proliferated in maternity wards, but later encroached on other parts of the hospitals and eventually escaped outside health care institutions, spreading within communities.[6] Penicillin, the miracle drug, wasn't working, and even newer and stronger medications like erythromycin and tetracycline were failing. Doctors everywhere were alarmed. The threat of bacterial infections had been declared vanquished a decade earlier, but it was suddenly back with a vengeance.

Before this frightening development, the medical world had fallen in love with antibiotics. Scientists learned that these wonder drugs not only cured lethal infections but prevented them from occurring. Pharmaceutical companies began putting antibiotics into various non-medicinal products, from ointments and toothpaste, to chewing gum and even lipstick.[7] Scientists discovered another astounding side effect of antibiotics' power: they made farm animals grow faster.

Like many seminal scientific breakthroughs, this discovery happened almost entirely by accident. Inspired by the mold-isolated penicillin, American pharmaceutical companies had been combing through various natural substances to find more miracle medications. They were particularly interested in soil, where many of these organisms live. Benjamin Duggar, a well-known botanist and plant pathologist who worked as a consultant for Lederle Laboratories, had been collecting soil samples from every place he traveled. In 1948, after scraping dirt at an experimental agronomy plot at the University of Missouri in Columbia, Duggar isolated a fungus that produced a bright yellow pigment that showed antibacterial qualities. In fact, it seemed to be so efficient that Duggar's "assistants and others were 'stealing' portions of the crude extracts to cure their colds," one paper stated.[8] (Today, we know that antibiotics can't cure viral colds, but they can cure the secondary bacterial infections that can develop following viral ones.) The colorful mold was christened *Streptomyces aureofaciens* and the antibiotic it oozed was named *aureomycin*, which later gave rise to the new class of drugs called *tetracyclines*.[9]

Coincidentally, in 1948, Lederle Laboratories was also delving into a different type of research—an agricultural endeavor aimed to produce healthier chickens. America's fast-growing, postwar population was hungry for protein, so meat producers were trying to raise the birds quickly and cheaply. To cut costs, they used soy feed, which proved not nutritious enough, leaving many chickens too skinny to consume. To boost growth, Lederle Laboratories worked to optimize the chicken chow with vitamins and other nutrients like liver extract. That process involved feeding several chicken flocks different diets and regularly weighing them. One of the flocks was put on a diet that included a by-product of aureomycin fermentation because it naturally had some vitamins in it—*S. aureofaciens* produces vitamin B12 as it grows.[10]

On Christmas Day of 1948, Thomas H. Jukes, the Lederle scientist in charge of the chickens' dietary welfare, weighed all his flocks, comparing their weight gain against each other. The chicks with plain soy did poorly, those supplemented with liver extract did better, but the ones that were pecking at the fermentation leftovers did amazingly well. They were, by far, the chubbiest of all. "I weighted the chicks on Christmas Day 1948 . . . ," Jukes wrote almost 40 forty years later in his recollections. "The chicks receiving aureomycin fermentation grew more rapidly than control chicks receiving liver extract."[11] Delighted with this development, Jukes and another collaborator submitted their findings to the American Chemical Society. A few months later, Lederle Laboratories started marketing aureomycin in animal feeds. "The decision was strongly opposed by the veterinarians at Lederle, but their wishes were abruptly denied," Jukes recalled.[12]

Fifteen months later, in April of 1950, the discovery was announced at the American Chemical Society's conference, becoming an instant sensation. "The golden-colored chemical lifesaving drug aureomycin of the group known as antibiotics has been found to be one of the greatest growth promoting substances so far to be discovered producing effects beyond those obtainable with any known vitamin," read the article by *New York Times* writer William L. Laurence, published the next morning.[13] Apparently, the substance, by then tried on various animals, fattened up hogs by 50 percent, with similar results on turkeys and chickens. Even better, it was incredibly cheap. Not only did it cost a mere thirty to forty cents per pound, but just five pounds of it added to a ton of animal fodder was enough to produce that spectacular growing effect.

Quoting the researchers, the article stated that the discovery is believed to "hold enormous long-range significance for the survival of the human race in the world of dwindling resources and expanding populations." Moreover, scientists thought aureomycin could be the perfect drug to treat undernourished, sickly children. "Clinical investigations on human subjects to check the possibility that aureomycin's hitherto unsuspected nutritional powers may also aid the growth of malnourished and undersized children in addition to extending the world's meat supply and decreasing its costs are now underway."[14] With that, antibiotics had firmly planted themselves in the American farming and food supply—for decades to come.

Not every scientist, however, was as excited about antibiotics. Some were already seeing, and cautioning about, the dark side of the drugs—the emerging resistance. After all, there were early signs—so early that they came before the medicines were even used. On December 28, 1940, before the first wonder drug had been given to a human, Ernst Chain, who later perfected the penicillin production with Howard Florey, and Edward Abraham, an Oxford University researcher, published a letter in the journal *Nature*,[15] stating that they observed the intestinal bacteria *E. coli* evolve an ability to resist penicillin. After several experiments, they decreed that this *E. coli* strain now possessed an enzyme that somehow inactivated the penicillin molecules. Moreover, they found that another bug, *Micrococcus luteus*, was able to interfere with penicillin too, albeit less expertly. They called the enzyme *penicillinase* but had yet to figure out how it worked. "The mechanism of the enzymatic inactivation of penicillin is being studied," they wrote.[16] Today, we know that the resistant bugs ooze out this enzyme akin to squids that squirt out ink. The penicillinase leaves the bacterial cell and degrades the penicillin molecules around it.[17]

Five years later, when Alexander Fleming accepted his Nobel Prize for discovering penicillin's powers, he cautioned that the careless and improper use of the drug would enable the germs to develop defenses. "The time may come when penicillin can be bought by anyone in the shops," he said presciently. "Then there is the danger that the ignorant man may easily underdose himself and by exposing his microbes to non-lethal quantities of the drug make them resistant. Here is a hypothetical illustration. Mr. X has a sore throat. He buys some penicillin and gives himself, not enough to kill the streptococci but enough to educate them to resist penicillin. He then infects his wife. Mrs. X gets pneumonia and is treated with penicillin. As the streptococci are now resistant to penicillin the treatment fails. Mrs. X dies. Who is primarily responsible for Mrs. X's death? Why Mr. X whose negligent use of penicillin changed the nature of the microbe."[18]

Little did Fleming know that this scenario wouldn't be limited to average citizens' negligent use of penicillin. That misuse would quickly become widespread, promoted, and bolstered by several powerful industries and the policymakers they influenced. For a long period of time, the scientists' warnings remained largely unheeded. The animal growers who fed antibiotics to their poultry and cattle, as well as the manufacturers who added antibiotics to skin creams, gums, and lipstick were doing exactly what scientists cautioned about—exposing the bugs to the drugs, letting them develop defenses.

Indiscriminately throwing antibiotics into the environment—by way of feeding them to farm animals or adding them to everyday products—puts selective pressures on the germs. The weakest die and the strongest survive. Some do so by spontaneous mutations, evolving genes that produce defensive enzymes or pump antibiotics out of their cells. Others may acquire antibiotic-resistant genes from their already evolved brethren through the phenomenon called *horizontal gene transfer*, in which two bacteria cozy up to each other, open up their cell walls, and trade their tricks via the so-called plasmids, snippets of genetic material. Plus, some resistant mutants may already exist in nature but are being suppressed by their faster-multiplying "cousins." If these dominant cousins turn out to be susceptible to antibiotics and die out, their resistant relatives can then proliferate unrestrained.

Whether or not the 1950s staph outbreak was caused or exacerbated by the growing use of antibiotics, it came to afflict not only the United States but also Canada, Great Britain, and Australia. The clinicians and researchers felt thrown back into the pre-antibiotic era. They were desperately trying to figure out how to beat this new, seemingly invincible germ.

The particular strain of S. aureus that was wreaking havoc in American hospitals in the 1950s was dubbed staph 80/81. The numbers had a very special meaning—and in some way an ironic one too. Long before genetic sequencing came of age, British scientists developed a different technique for typifying bacteria—meaning identifying the exact strain of staph, E. coli, or other germs. To typify the specific bacteria strain, they would use a set of different phages, each with a unique number assigned. They would seed a petri dish with the bacteria in question and sic the phages onto it. Depending on what phages lysed it, the bacterial strain would get that number attached to its name. In the case of the 1950s staphylococcus outbreak, phages 80 and 81 lysed the resistant strain of the S. aureus, so it became known as staph 80/81.[19]

The irony was that while doctors saw that the phages dissolved the bacteria under their very eyes, they didn't think of phages as therapeutics—only as diagnostic tools. They might have been able to see the phages' "tailwork" under the microscopes—by then, electronic microscopes offered enough resolution—but they didn't consider them medicines. Whether because phage preparations had been discredited in prior decades or because they were forgotten altogether, American doctors did not view phages as curative agents.

Instead, doctors developed an entirely different plan of attack. They tapped into staph's territorial nature, essentially fighting fire with fire. Author Maryn McKenna tells this story in her book, Superbug: The Fatal Menace of MRSA. Two physician researchers,

Heinz Eichenwald and Henry Shinefield, were working on the 1950s outbreak in the New York Hospital and noticed that the staph 80/81 wasn't the only strain present on the battlefield. There was another one, named 502a, which, unlike its vicious 80/81 relative, would peacefully dwell in the nose, throat, and skin of humans without causing any harm. Eichenwald and Shinefield noticed that babies who carried the 502a strain in and on themselves didn't fall ill with 80/81. Apparently, the 502a multiplied faster, pushing out its competitor before it could colonize the newborns. Eichenwald and Shinefield began giving babies drops of the 502a strain within their first hour of life—seeding the "nicer" staph into their noses and umbilical cords. Nine out of ten "seeded" babies wouldn't contract the 80/81 strain, and when they went home, they spread the beneficial staph to their families. The results were so striking that Shinefield began traveling to other hospitals around the country, seeding babies with the protective bug, saving lives, and curtailing the outbreaks.[20]

The staph 80/81 epidemic lasted for about ten years and then mysteriously began to wane. By 1963, the number of newborn and adult infections decreased.[21] It could be that the harmless, fast-growing 502a strain colonized enough humans, or perhaps that methicillin—a new and improved version of penicillin that the penicillinase enzyme couldn't shred—helped extinguish it. "The reason for the decline of phage-type 80/81 S. aureus is unknown," one article wrote, "but its dominance as a human pathogen ended a few years after methicillin was introduced as a treatment for infections caused by penicillin-resistant organisms."[22]

This long battle taught Western pharmacologists that more, better, and stronger antibiotics were needed. Over time, the concept of fighting staph with staph was abandoned—it turned out that the 502a strain could cause infections in some people. The only way to keep up with the evolving bugs was to keep evolving defenses against them. And so American pharmaceutical companies continued their quest for more powerful antibiotics, in a perpetual race against nature.

The race was, and still is, brutal. Just one look at the antibiotic development timeline makes it clear that humans never stood a chance of winning the microbial war. We were merely playing catch-up, sometimes managing to beat the bugs by a few years.[23] Tetracycline was introduced in 1950, but shigella learned to fight it off by 1959. Gentamicin arrived in 1967 and vancomycin in 1972, but enterococcus evolved to defeat the medications in 1979 and 1988, respectively, becoming the infamous VRE.[24] When, after years of development, linezolid was released to tackle VRE in 2000—at the same time Sandro was fruitlessly trying to get money to develop phage therapy—it lost its efficacy within four years. Some staph strains, already resistant to certain antibiotics, evaded linezolid even earlier.[25] But the most striking example of this exasperating battle was levofloxacin. The pneumococcus bacteria became resistant to it the same year it was brought to market.[26] The bugs took far less time to evolve their defenses than we took to develop ours. If they had a consciousness, they would have laughed in our faces.

The methicillin triumph over S. aureus was equally short-lived. As early as 1961, while the hospital staph cases were beginning to decline, scientists in the United Kingdom already saw some S. aureus strains developing resistance to antibiotics. Right before their eyes, the resourceful germs were evolving into the soon-to-be infamous methicillin-resistant S. aureus, or MRSA.[27,28,29] It was only a matter of time before this resistant strain would begin to traverse the world.

MRSA took some time to strike, but cases began to rise in the 1970s. In sterile hospital settings, where its natural competitors were conveniently extinguished, MRSA could settle down comfortably, traveling through wards on equipment and even on staffers, who became unwitting unsusceptible carriers—and then attack a vulnerable patient who had just undergone surgery. Overpowering such patients' weakened immune systems, MRSA caused pneumonia, osteomyelitis, lung abscesses, enterocolitis, and sepsis, sometimes resulting in death. Patients took endless courses of antibiotics, only to see the infections return again and again, for months and even years. And even when they managed to finally beat it, they were often left physically and emotionally devastated—and facing massive hospital bills.

The Soviet Union, relatively isolated from the world by the Iron Curtain, wasn't immune to MRSA. There, the golden staph also wreaked havoc in maternity wards, hospitals, and communities. As a country, the USSR was even more vulnerable to it, because of the often crowded and unhygienic living conditions. But the Soviets used varied defenses. They never abandoned living medicines in favor of synthesized ones. While Western pharmaceutical companies were trying to outrun bacteria with increasingly powerful and often toxic molecules, the Soviet scientists made nature an ally. And by 1970, they had all but found the cure for MRSA.

HUNTING DOWN THE GOLDEN DEVIL

At age twenty-five, Avtandil Chkeidze was dying. His health had been steadily declining for a decade, his body progressively losing its strength and vigor. Over the past ten years, the *Staphylococcus aureus* bacteria made his body its permanent home, invading his blood and spreading to his internal organs. Chkeidze lived with chronic systemic sepsis, a rare form of the disease.

It all started when Chkeidze was a teenager. He developed a bad case of acne—an infection caused by *S. aureus*—the golden staph. Most teens with this problem outgrow it after a few years. Chkeidze didn't. Rather than eventually easing up, *furuncles* and their clusters, called *carbuncles*, began to appear everywhere on his skin. His face, chest, and back were covered with an oozing rash that sometimes developed into ulcers with festering centers. Chkeidze's father, a doctor, bandaged his son every day. A military medic, he had tried every known antibiotic with little effect. The golden killer that invaded his son deflected the highest level of Soviet defense, erythromycin, with the same ease our MRSA shrugs off methicillin. Usually, if sepsis doesn't respond to antibiotics, it kills within days or weeks, causing high fevers and organ failure. But in Chkeidze's case, the bug settled in, eating through his body inch by inch and day by day.

It also robbed the young man of his ability to practice medicine. Following his father's footsteps, Chkeidze had studied to be a doctor and, despite battling the nasty infection, earned his diploma. But as his health worsened, the Soviet equivalent of the medical board rescinded his license, concerned that he would spread his infection to his patients.

Chkeidze's case was unique, but the threat of the antibiotic-resistant *S. aureus* was not. In the 1970s, the golden staph became a significant concern across the country. By then, antibiotics were common, and doctors prescribed them regularly. Just as in Western countries, that practice led to the development of resistant, mutant strains.

Certain Soviet socioeconomic conditions fueled the *S. aureus* spread. One of them was the construction of the Baikal–Amur Mainline, or BAM—a 2,687-mile-long railway in the USSR's far east, stretching through half of Siberia all the way to the eastern shore. The BAM was strategically important for the economy, so in their classic approach, the Soviet authorities called out to the selfless devotion of the country's young to build the railroad for their motherland. The idealistic enthusiasts came, but the government hadn't created the proper working conditions.

The BAM builders languished in squalor and permafrost. Some lived in tents, where the temperature never rose above the freezing point. Others lived in barely heated barracks. There was no hot water and in some cases no running water. In some places, there were no sewers, and in others, they leaked. Coming home from a hard day of physical labor, workers couldn't take showers or launder clothes, often staying unwashed for days and weeks. Their accumulating sweat clogged their skin pores, allowing infections to settle in, quickly taking hold in cuts and lacerations. When they could wash, they often shared the same towels, spreading staph around.[30] Many were covered in furuncles. In some, skin infection would spread to bones, causing osteomyelitis. From there, it could easily make it into the bloodstream, resulting in sepsis.

David Shrayer-Petrov, a Soviet doctor and microbiologist who was sent from Moscow to Siberia to tame the outbreaks, documented the devastation in his memoir, *Hunting Down the Golden Devil*, and also in his science monograph, *Staphylococcus Disease in the Soviet Union: Epidemiology and Response to a National Epidemic*. One of the BAM locations, called Nizhneangarsk, was in particularly dire shape. "The Nizhneangarsk hospital has 100 beds as well as surgical, therapeutic, obstetric, and pediatric wards. Staff visitors and patients moved freely from one department to another, contributing to an uninhibited exchange of bacteria and disease. The streets of Nizhneangarsk were full of stray dogs, garbage and rats. The town's residents lived in wooden huts with no running water, plumbing or sewer system." Nizhneangarsk's epidemiology station was similarly housed in a wooden hut with a lab equipped with only a microscope, refrigerator, and incubator.[31]

When winter relented and spring arrived, it often made things worse. "The melting of snow flooded the streets with fecal masses

and even when there were outhouses there was no sewage purification systems," Shrayer-Petrov writes. "Because of these conditions
Nizhneangarsk became a pathogenic cesspool for staphylococcal
disease and other infections."[32] Furuncles and carbuncles spread
between workers like wildfire.

The BAM's "cesspool" wasn't self-contained. Even if BAM
workers managed to avoid getting sick or recovered, when they
went back home, they carried the staph with them, spreading it
far and wide. The golden killer hitched a ride on their skin, their
clothes, and their boots. It traveled cross-country on the trains
they took, seeping into sheets they slept on and towels they used.
Once they arrived home, they brought it into their houses and the
houses of others too. And while some strains still succumbed to
antibiotics, others did no more.

Doctors began to see people whose initially minor skin infections would progress into systemic ones, putting people on life
support. Some patients developed them after routine surgical
procedures, in large part because doctors who treated them were
often the unwitting carriers. In one case in Moscow, more than
half of the staff harbored staph, and nearly half of them harbored
the infamous 80/81 strain. In the Siberian city of Barnaul, over 87
percent of medical personnel in a pediatric hospital, as well as the
children's mothers, carried it.[33]

In such favorable conditions, the staph would firmly take hold
on the skin lesions of diabetics, ignoring topical antibiotics and
waiting for an opportune moment to slip into the bloodstream. In
Moscow, the antibiotic-resistant *S. aureus* ran rampant in the neo-
natal care units to the point that it became unsafe to have a baby
in a hospital. The staph attacked the newborns' unprepared immune systems and stymied their growth. Pale, limp, and weak, the
infected infants couldn't gain weight and missed developmental
milestones, and some died. Some women took the risk of traveling

to other cities—on planes, trains, and automobiles—to give birth in distant hospitals. Others decided to deliver at home. The Soviet medical system desperately needed an antibiotic alternative.

It turned out that Tbilisi's Bacteriological Institute, founded by Eliava and at the time called the Institute of Vaccines and Serums, had one in the works.

By the 1970s, the institute was producing several tons of intestinal bacteriophage preparations a day. It was also producing loads of vials for skin infections. But the phage preparations needed to treat the systemic infections had to be administered intravenously so they could reach all organs—and those remained unattainable so far. Even d'Hérelle in his last book noted that phage given intravenously sometimes worked and sometimes resulted in drastic and dangerous side effects, spiking high fevers or causing terrible headaches. These symptoms of shock signaled to scientists that the body was having an allergic reaction, and it wasn't clear how to avoid that result.

Today, we know that the deleterious effects are caused by various chemicals present in the lysate—the resulting brew of the phage-bacterial war. Besides phages, lysates contain shreds of dead microbes, their broken DNA, pieces of their cell walls, and gooey cytoplasm. It is not a clean and salubrious solution but a noxious battleground goo. "First you take a deadly bacterium and you grow it in a culture, then add a little bit of phage and go away for a few hours," explains Ryland Young, professor emeritus at Texas A&M University, who spent over forty years studying bacteriophages and their prey. "When you come back there's this soup of phage, broken bacteria, its DNA and the shreds of its busted cells." And not all bacteria are even dead yet. That soup may also contain the products of bacterial metabolism, which can be toxic to humans. Plus, many bacteria have certain molecules on their cellular walls called *lipopolysaccharides*, which our immune system recognizes as foreign and therefore also toxic, so once it sees them, it may go into overdrive. Scientists use the word *endotoxin* to describe them, and in some bacterial species, these molecules cover the bugs' entire outer coats. "If you put a lot of endotoxins in your blood, you go into shock," explains Young. "So if you have a lot of dead bacterial cells and you inject all that into the patient's bloodstream, you're going to kill your patient. You have to get rid of it or bring it down at least to a certain level."

The phage production team purified all phage preparations by passing the solutions through various filters and using centrifuges to separate the parts. For the intestinal, wound, and skin applications, that level of purification was enough. But the intravenous administration needed a cleaner solution. Teimuraz Chanishvili, Nina's uncle and Sandro Sulakvelidze's future PhD advisor, had devoted close to twenty years to solving this problem. He believed that in the case of MRSA, patients' allergic reactions were caused by the leftover products of bacterial metabolism. *S. aureus*, for example, can ooze out a whole list of different toxins as it multiplies before becoming phage food itself. Chanishvili thought he could make *S. aureus* produce fewer toxins by feeding it a different type of broth. So he decided to put the golden devil "on a diet," explains Nina Chanishvili.

Rather than feeding it a rich and nourishing beef broth, Chanishvili grew the bug on a meager subsistence of a saline-based solution synthesized to be very nutrient poor. Just as d'Hérelle had once changed the medium on which the yersinia bacteria grew, Chanishvili did so for staph. Bacteria that grew in such "starving" conditions weren't able to release much protein, which resulted in a cleaner preparation.

Chanishvili and his team spent years perfecting their cleaned-up therapy in the lab. They tested it in mice with no reaction. They infused it to rabbits with no adverse effects. Eventually, they administered it to healthy human volunteers, who also tolerated it well. Yet they hadn't made the leap from the healthy humans to sepsis-stricken patients struggling to survive. And that's where Chkeidze came in.

A trained physician himself, the young man read about Chanishvili's work and asked his father to reach out. By then, Chkeidze walked with a cane like a much older man and required frequent rests. He had been treated with various antibiotics at the country's best hospitals—in Moscow, in Leningrad, in Tbilisi. Most recently, his father took him to the Skin Diseases Clinic at the Military Medical Academy in Leningrad—to no avail. "I have nothing to lose, and I want to try it," Chkeidze said. His father and Chanishvili enlisted Professor Vakhtang Bochorishvili from Tbilisi's Sepsis Center as the attending physician, and the young man was admitted to the hospital as a willing guinea pig.

Every two days, Chkeidze received phage transfusions, which once again proved that they could do miracles when all else fails. Three days later, he already felt better. His ulcers began to close with normal skin epithelium. New rashes stopped developing. He had more energy. On day four, he tossed away his cane. By day five, he felt like a mischievous, fun-craving twenty-five-year-old. One of his friends was having a birthday, so Chkeidze, still officially checked in to the sepsis ward, decided to attend. "A group of friends 'kidnapped' him from the hospital," Nina Chanishvili shares the story. "He climbed out the window and went to the party." Later that day, or perhaps in the wee hours of the morning, he surreptitiously slipped back in—a man who couldn't walk without a cane just a week prior. After the seventh transfusion, he felt good, was discharged, and went home. He reinstated his medical license, practiced medicine, got married, and had healthy children. The staff never returned.[34]

Encouraged by this result, the phage-and-physician duo began treating other chronic sepsis patients who ran out of the antibiotic options. Most of them experienced little to no side effects. Some developed fevers but usually not too high, and they recovered remarkably quickly—often within days. One of the patients, a thirty-two-year-old woman with acute sepsis, was sixteen weeks pregnant. On day three of phage transfusions, her fever dropped—and months later, she delivered a healthy baby.

On April 11, 1979, Soviet health authorities gave several major hospitals in Moscow and Tbilisi permission to try the new treatment in clinical trials. After the intravenous staphylococcal phage preparation was successfully tested on nearly one thousand people, the institute began mass-producing it. "They made eight hundred to one thousand liters of this phage a year," says Nina Chanishvili. "They shipped it all over the country."

Staph bacteria can be highly variable, so not every phage would devour every bug. To circumvent that, Chanishvili's team developed a polyvalent phage cocktail. Overall, the staphylococcal phage treatment was so successful that in February 1983, it was approved for treating children, including newborns in the maternity wards still plagued by the golden killer. Doctors who administered the treatment to the pale and limp infants watched them change color and gain strength before their very eyes. Their cheeks went pink. Their eyes opened. They began eating and gained weight in just a few days. The living medicines had breathed them back to life.

The staph cocktail also helped to tame the BAM epidemic. Shrayer-Petrov and his colleagues used it to hunt down and exterminate the golden devil from the hospitals and barracks of Nizhneangarsk. "Polyvalent staphylococcal bacteriophage was applied with wads, bandages, sprinkles and lotions during washing of

lesions and abscesses (following pus removal) as well as intravenously and with intratracheal administration and intramuscular injections," Shrayer-Petrov wrote. "Soon patients' overall conditions
improved, staphylococci stopped growing, wounds were without
pus and began to granulate." Preoccupied with curing as many
people as possible, Shrayer-Petrov did not keep a control group,
but the cocktail worked against 90 percent of staph isolated from
patients and cleared infections within about a week of treatment.[35]

Besides keeping BAM outbreaks in check, phages also kept the
Soviet military recruits healthy and functioning. In the USSR, the
draft was compulsory—the majority of young men had to serve
for at least two years once they turned eighteen. Only students at
the top universities in the country were exempted. Their brains
were deemed more important than their military prowess, so instead of two years of military training, they were allowed to serve
for just a few weeks a year.

The draftees usually were shipped off to distant locations.
Those from Moscow suburbs would be sent to the bases in the
Soviet Central Asia. Those from the far east would find themselves
on the western borders. They would also get mixed and matched
with other recruits from all over the country. The army's assign-
ments intentionally served to forge a unified nation that spoke one
language: Russian. But changing geographic locales and mingling
with new people meant being exposed to unfamiliar microbes that
invariably caused intestinal and other problems. With barracks
life and outdoor latrines, familiar scourges like dysentery and E.
coli immediately reared their heads. The army used the institute's
phage preparations for treatment and prophylaxis.

Phages were also used in agriculture to fight bacteria-caused
plant and animal disease. In the West, this was being accomplished
with antibiotics. But in the Soviet Union, antibiotics were still

expensive to produce and were primarily used for treating humans rather than feeding farm animals or adding them to everyday products. The outcomes of phage treatments on farms differed from those produced by Western antibiotics. The antibiotics killed weaker germs, allowing the vicious ones to develop. Phages did what they normally did in nature—they attacked their prey and kept up with the bugs' evolution. The Soviet Union needed phages, and while a few other institutions across the country grew some too, Tbilisi's Institute of Vaccines and Serums was the largest producer by far.

The 1980s were the institute's golden era. If Eliava and d'Hérelle could see what their vision blossomed into, they would have been proud. About eight hundred people worked in the production department alone.[36] On the first floor of the manufacturing building, they cooked up thousands of gallons of broth daily from beef and other ingredients. That soup was pumped onto the third floor through pipes and loaded into massive incubator machines, each of which held over 130 gallons. Every morning, the upstairs crew loaded up bacterial cultures and let them feast and procreate in the soup. Later on, they added phages. Once the phages grew and reproduced, the staff harvested and filtered them. The curative viruses were packaged into vials, which, until the 1970s, was done by hand—a regular worker filled five hundred to six hundred, and an expert one could manage one thousand per shift. Later, there came dispensing machines. Eventually, the institute began producing some phages in a dry form as powder pressed into tablets. They stayed inactive until consumed.[37] Throughout those years, the institute produced thousands of pills and vials daily and shipped them all over the country. After developing the intravenous staph phage, it was on course to develop more living medicines and save more lives.

But then, on the chilly Monday of March 11, 1985, after the

rapid-fire deaths of three Soviet leaders in less than three years—Leonid Brezhnev, Yuri Andropov, and Konstantin Chernenko—Mikhail Gorbachev became the country's next general secretary. No one could foresee what would happen next.

9

Phages Endangered

The bullet shells were everywhere. They carpeted the entire road that weaved around the base of Mount Mtatsminda—the Holy Mountain on top of which rose Tbilisi's TV tower. They rustled underneath people's feet like fallen leaves in autumn. After a few days of fighting, the insurgents who rebelled against Georgia's president, Zviad Gamsakhurdia, took over the TV tower, leaving behind overturned trucks and buildings spattered with bullet holes. Periodically, they fired from the mountaintop. Walking along the battered streets, Nina Chanishvili and her mother jammed themselves toward the side of the mountain to avoid being hit from above. They were bringing food to the two elderly women who lived in the midst of the battlefield and couldn't leave their home for days. "We brought them bread and canned food because canned food was all we had," Chanishvili recalls. "They cried when they saw us."

Like most Georgians in 1992, Chanishvili was a seasoned survivor. Tbilisi was chaotic and dysfunctional. Electricity was rare. Homes and buildings went without heat for months. In winter, people slept in coats and hats. They set up fires in their courtyards to cook meals, which they often shared with their neighbors, knowing that the next day their neighbors might feed them if they ran out of sustenance. The lines for food were enormous—five hundred people would instantly queue up at the sight of a chicken, fish, or egg delivery because they often hadn't seen any for months.

"It was a very hard time, but we felt that we all were in the same boat, so we had to help each other," Chanishvili says. "And we kept our spirits high."

Next came the exceptionally snowy winter that paralyzed the city. There was no mass transit. There was still no heat. But Georgians stood strong. "There was no bread, but the theater was working!" Chanishvili recalls. The actors staged *A Midsummer Night's Dream* by William Shakespeare. "It was freezing inside, so the audience wore winter coats," she says. "But the actors flew around the stage wrapped in transparent tunics. I was so impressed by them!"

Tbilisians had learned to live in the new post-Soviet reality, amid the intermittent violence of Georgia's civil war. One night, Chanishvili woke up to see the red traces of bullets outside her window. "Should I get up and hide?" she wondered. So many people were being hit by strays during those turbulent months that hiding would have been wise. But she was so exhausted from a lack of sleep, a shortage of food, being cold, and the constant struggle to survive that she couldn't move. *To hell with this. Whatever happens, happens*, she thought, falling back asleep. The kids were safe, and that was all that mattered. Chanishvili lived together with her mother, sister, and uncle as one big family. Her nephews' beds had long been moved into the middle of the house, into the hallways with no windows so that no stray bullets could find them.[1]

People weren't the only ones living under constant threat. Biological specimens were endangered too. When electricity began to shut off, thousands of samples cultivated and stored at the Eliava Institute, now proudly bearing the name of its founder, were in peril. While therapeutic phage cocktails can stay active for some time at room temperature, many specific samples were made to be stored in freezers long term. And it wasn't just phages that were threatened. The bacterial samples that scientists used to feed their living medicines, as well as to keep track of emerging pathogens, were endangered too.[2]

This was a problem of huge magnitude, with far-reaching implications. Over the years, the institute gathered a massive collection of bacterial strains and their predators. In 1967, the Soviet minister of health issued a law requiring that all pathogenic bacterial strains found in any corner of the country—which sprawled across much of Eurasia occupying over eight million square miles—be sent to the Eliava Institute. The Soviet republics complied, and the institute received forty-two thousand strains over time. As they arrived, the bugs were examined, cataloged, and fed to their predators to identify which phage cocktails would destroy them. This information was recorded so that if a particular strain caused an outbreak anywhere in the Soviet empire, Tbilisi scientists could fetch the appropriate phage vials from their library and begin growing them en masse. Processing the forty-two thousand strains was an exhausting effort that took months, if not years, but at the end, the Eliava Institute was well equipped to fight many deadly germs.[3]

The original project morphed into an ongoing effort to stay one step ahead of the ever-evolving bugs. After the initial cataloging was done, Eliava scientists continued receiving samples from across the USSR. "Every new strain that came from some place in the Soviet Union came to us," says Zemphira Alavidze, who had led the Laboratory of Morphology and Biology of Phages before Georgia separated from the Soviet Union. Over eighty years old now, Alavidze works for a private medical company. "Our institute tested if we had phages that were active against these strains. If some strains were resistant to our existing production phages, they were sent to my lab. We had to either find phages active against these strains or cultivate them," she says—according to d'Hérelle's original approach. "Once we had these active phages, we passed them to the production team so they could be added to the existing cocktails and be mass-produced. That's how we kept our phage medicines current at all times." This ongoing biological vigilance was unmatched by any other in the world.[4]

This effort reveals an interesting ideological perspective, different from Western approaches. The American pharmaceutical industry hoped that every new antibiotic would last long enough that the health care system and society wouldn't have to worry for a while. Alas, the germs tended to evolve faster than expected and put doctors on the defensive. Soviet scientists, however, accepted the fact that they would never be able to lower their guard and would always have to be on the lookout for novel strains. The cost of that effort was no doubt substantial, but it allowed them to be better prepared to fight the worst pathogens. Neither did Soviet scientists put their entire research faith into molecules that were hard to find and expensive to bring to market. Instead, they would sic one organism on another and pick the winners. It was much easier than trying to outrun nature, and in the end, it created an unparalleled collection of pathogens and their destroyers.

That collection, along with knowledge of the operations and procedures needed to sustain it, was absolutely unique. Now, it was threatened because there were no resources to keep it alive.

With no heat and no electricity, hundreds of samples cultivated and stored at the Eliava Institute were going to perish. To save the samples, scientists who still had electricity in their apartments divvied up phage vials and boxes, packed them up into bags, and took them home. "My home was in the part of the city where some government officials lived, so we still had power," recalls Mzia Kutateladze, back then a lab technician and now the institute's director. "I put as much as I could—a bunch of boxes in my bag—took them home and stuffed them into my freezer, where they stayed for a while." At the time, her freezer, as well as her colleagues' freezers, had plenty of space because food was scarce. Some scientists went back and forth multiple times, ferrying living medicines to safe locations via poorly running public transport that often was so packed that people hung out of the doors, holding on to whatever they could.[5]

In winter, when the temperature inside the institute hovered around zero degrees centigrade, preserving specimens was a little easier—they could be stored at "room temperature," at least for a while. Members of the institute staff kept coming to work even in those impossible conditions, conducting their lab meetings dressed in winter coats, scarves, and hats. "We were frozen, but our phages were doing fine," Chanishvili quips.

Saving bacterial samples was much more difficult. Phages were therapeutic agents, not only harmless but beneficial for people, so they could be carried outside the institute, onto buses and trains— and into one's home. The hazardous bacterial pathogens, which were needed for research, vaccine production, and phage preparations, could not leave the campus. And so the absolutely unique biological library of pathogenic microbes gathered from the vast reaches of the Eurasian continent over decades was irreparably lost. "We couldn't take them home, couldn't carry them in mass transit, couldn't put them in our freezers next to food," says Kutateladze. Some of them were extremely dangerous. "So we saved what we could. We lost our bacterial collection, but we were lucky to preserve our phages."[6]

To survive, some scientists turned to more practical work, such as diagnosing and treating disease. Alavidze and her colleagues began producing therapeutic phages to treat those wounded in battle during the armed conflicts that shook Georgia, including the so-called Abkhazian war, sparked by the Abkhazian ethnic minority's desire to separate into their own country. Fighters carried bottles with them into the battles and sprayed phages on wounds, which reportedly decreased infections dramatically.

Amid the chaos, Chanishvili was invited to spend a year doing phage research in the lab of Lucien Caro at the University of Geneva—the same institution where Giorgi Eliava started his microbiology ascent eight decades prior. "It was a hard decision," Chanishvili recalls. She felt wrong leaving her family behind during such difficult times. She was taking care of her now-elderly uncle as well as her nephew, because her sister fell ill with hepatitis after giving birth. And she was taking care of whatever still functioned at the institute.

After a long deliberation, she finally decided to go. Caro had sent her a Swiss Air ticket, but the only way to fly to Geneva was through Moscow, where planes from Tbilisi almost never flew anymore. After much turmoil, Chanishvili managed to get onto a Moscow-bound plane. She was lucky to have a seat because many passengers flew standing on the overcrowded plane. Halfway through the flight, the plane had to stop in Sochi, a city in Russia's south, because it ran out of fuel. At last, with five dollars in her pocket (the accumulation of several months of her salary) and a coat borrowed from a relative, Chanishvili landed in Geneva. The research was exciting, but she remained exhausted from prior stress, worries about her kin, the language barrier, and the continuous culture shock. She felt foreign in the posh European city and, in a way, was relieved to return to the struggling Tbilisi. "In Geneva, I was always an outsider, but here, I was home, and we were all in it together."

By then, the era of the so-called privatization was moving in. With no more government support, all previously state-owned establishments had to learn to fend for themselves. The Eliava

Institute's phage factory employed more people in production than it did researchers, so it was deemed a business—and moved under the auspices of the Ministry of Production. "And then the ministry declared that everything will be privatized and so we were privatized the same way as shoemaking or electronic assembly," Chanishvili says.

To make a living, scientists had to find practical uses for their expertise and turn their laboratories into private enterprises, offering either treatment or diagnostic services, or producing phage-based medicines. One after another, autonomous cooperatives split off from the institute, each renting its own space, paying its own bills, and trying to survive as best it could. "The ten production plants, which used to make a gamut of therapeutic and diagnostic phages during the Soviet time, became ten private companies, each trying to survive on their own," Chanishvili says.

Alavidze, whose Soviet-era work was closely connected to the local clinics and hospitals, began producing phages for them. Instead of the big production vats that grew enough phages to supply the entire USSR, they went small. "We made little batches and sent them to burn centers, surgery, urology, dermatology," Alavidze says. It was a way to make money, pay the bills, and keep the process going. "The main goal was to preserve the collection of phages. If we didn't do this, we could lose the entire production process. Many labs did close. But we came every day, and we preserved it."

Sometime during the chaos of the 1990s, American phage researcher Elizabeth Kutter from Evergreen State College visited the institute and gave a lecture. Although she had spent her whole career studying the genetics of a particular phage called T-4, she had never heard of living medicines. She wanted to see the production labs and learn about the process. When she left, she was intrigued.

"I think it opened some doors for us," says Alavidze—Kutter became one of the institute's first Western supporters, advocating for the phages internationally. "She organized phage conferences in Seattle," says Kutateladze. "She always made new bridges for us with other scientists, and she helped us get grants." One of the early grants, which came from the Hungarian-American businessman and philanthropist George Soros, helped the institute preserve its phage collection. "Every little bit helped."

The breakthrough came one day in 1996, when Chanishvili's phone rang. On the other line was American journalist Peter Radetsky, a writer and contributing editor to *Discover* magazine. Radetsky was no stranger to viruses. Just a few years earlier, he had published the book *The Invisible Invaders: The Story of the Emerging Age of Viruses*, full of stories about scientists who tracked them down, from Louis Pasteur to the discoverers of HIV. Somehow this writing journey led him to the struggling Eliava Institute, which saw viruses from the opposite perspective. As the conversation progressed, Radetsky asked how the institute was surviving in the post-Soviet era. "I can't possibly explain this to you on the phone," Chanishvili said. "We haven't been paid salaries for several months. We don't have food. We don't have electricity. You'd have to come to understand it, and you'd have to see it to believe it." Radetsky, who was no stranger to traveling off the beaten path, took her answer as an invitation and hopped on a plane.

He met Nina. He spoke to her uncle Teimuraz. He listened to stories of the institute's old glory. He toured what was left of the campus. The sight of the devastation was so depressing that Nina thought Radetsky wasn't even sure how to write about it. "Let's see what we can do with it," she remembers him saying before he got on the plane home.

The article came out shortly thereafter. It was an objective story that illuminated the struggling institute and the looming loss of the important scientific knowledge. "The sprawling campus on the bank of the Mtkvari River is crumbling. . . . Corridors are gloomy, doors are padlocked, windows groan and slam in the wind," Radetsky wrote. He lamented the world's ignorance. "The West [is] increasingly desperate for new treatments against bacterial diseases, and Tbilisi's Bacteriophage Institute, the font of such treatments, [is] increasingly desperate to just survive."[7] The grandfather of bacteriophages would certainly relate, Radetsky added. "Félix d'Hérelle would have appreciated the irony," he wrote. "He may have appreciated it, that is, when he wasn't railing against the rest of the world for not paying attention.[8]

And the world finally did.

One of the first people to pay attention was American venture capitalist Caisey Harlingten, a former stockbroker who was now looking for investment opportunities. He read the article flying home from Toronto to Seattle and was instantly intrigued. Radetsky included independent experts' opinions on whether phage therapies could possibly receive the FDA approval. There were skeptics, but also some supporters, Elizabeth Kutter among them. She acknowledged that phages would be a hard sell for the FDA but that the question was worth exploring. Harlingten read it as a great opportunity the world had missed so far. He called Kutter and asked if she'd come with him to Tbilisi. She said yes. And then he called Nina Chanishvili.

Shortly thereafter, Harlingten landed in Georgia not only with Kutter but with his whole family in tow. He was genuinely enthusiastic and compassionate. The sight of researchers discussing scientific matters wrapped in winter coats, scarves, and gloves made a deep impression on him, so he immediately bought several heaters for the institute. He gave Chanishvili money to set up a new laboratory in an abandoned building. He decided to form the Georgia Research Institute and asked Nina to lead the creation of the new company. But he also needed a different figure in the mix. He wanted someone who could split their time between America and

Tbilisi, someone who could understand the nuances of Georgian culture and the complexities of the FDA's inner workings. Someone who could wear both hats with equal ease, depending on the day and the continent.

"I think I know just the right person," Nina said.

10

A Georgian in Maryland

Sandro's first few months in America were full of excitement. He found Baltimore's Inner Harbor spectacular. He thought an ATM was nothing short of a miracle. His first trip to a supermarket was a revelation.

"I am looking for a store where I can buy some bread and cheese," he told Glenn Morris's wife, Deborah, who offered to drive him to go food shopping because he had no car.

"What kind of bread and what kind of cheese?" she asked.

"Just any bread and cheese," Sandro responded, unaccustomed to options. In Tbilisi, he'd enter a bread store and grab whatever loaf was available. And then he'd ask for half a kilo of cheese and the salesperson would reach for *the cheese*—the one and only type delivered that day—and hack off a chunk. When Sandro walked up to a cheese counter in an American supermarket, he was dumbfounded. "I was awed. I had no idea what to buy."

But as weeks went by, Sandro began to miss home. Georgia has a famously communal culture that means one is never alone for long. Sandro grew up with his three cousins as if they were siblings. They lived in the same building, went to the same school, and spent summers in the same cottage in the countryside. The home was always full of people—aunts, uncles, cousins twice- and thrice-removed. Sandro's father, Levan, played piano and sang romances, so guests came often. And then there were the neighbors. When kids got too loud, the elderly lady next door would ring the bell, but instead of chastising them, she brought the *khachapuri* cheese breads, fresh off the pan. "You must be very tired from all that activity," she would say kindly, holding the steaming plate. "Why don't you take a break and have some food?" Sandro missed that level of human connection.

Career-wise, he had everything he could dream of at Morris's lab. He enjoyed the most sophisticated equipment he had ever worked with. He had all the reagents he could wish for. He could investigate nearly any scientific questions he wanted. But he was lonely. He missed his home, his family, and his friends. He missed his fiancée, Nino.

Even when Morris's fellowship letter first arrived, he had experienced pangs of doubt. Was he doing the right thing, going away? Could he really leave his elderly father behind, all alone, while the country was falling apart? Was it a selfish thing to do? On a warm summer day, in the family's countryside home, he told his cousins about the offer. They were happy for his success, yet sad to see him go. It was unimaginable that someone you saw every day of your life would be gone for almost a year.[1]

Sandro's father told him to go. So did his uncle Vazha. A hardcore scientist himself, Vazha had done research in the United States. He knew what Sandro would be missing if he didn't go. "It's a different world," he told his nephew. "It's the world of opportunities. Don't let that chance pass you by!" Sandro, who always felt he had a special bond with his uncle, took his advice. Nine months, after all, would fly by.

Nine months indeed flew by, but his comparisons of different yersinias' pathogenic threats were so interesting that Morris wanted him to keep working. When Sandro first came from Tbilisi, he brought several yersinia strains from Georgia, which naturally dwelled in soil or animal feces and could be a ticking time bomb. Science knew little about them. Were they deadly? Did they respond to antibiotics? Could an outbreak cause a pandemic one day? Morris's father was a missionary, so he grew up in Asia and knew too well that infectious disease could simmer in wildlife for ages—and then spill over to humans. When Morris and Sandro saw their mice dying from what they thought to be a mild bug, they knew there was more to study. "If we can find you a research position, would you stay for another year?" Morris asked.

At first, Sandro turned down the offer. Nino and he had agreed to marry as soon as he was back. His job as a laboratory director was still waiting for him. But then he spoke to Nino and reconsidered. "If I can bring Nino over, I would stay," he told Morris.

Morris pulled together some resources and offered Sandro a $20,000 salary for a yearlong research position. With that money, Sandro could afford to rent a small apartment of his own and bring Nino along. The University of Maryland issued an official visa request for Nino, and Sandro flew back to Tbilisi to get married and start the paperwork for her to come to Maryland.

His visit was bittersweet. He was happy to see everyone he left behind—Nino, his father, his cousins, and his dog. Yet the country was in such bad shape, it was unsafe to live there. Armed conflicts and poverty devastated the city and society. Buildings were pockmarked with bullet holes, windows were broken, and crime was rampant. Armed with weapons that recent conflicts made easy to get, criminals hijacked cars in broad daylight, broke into homes, and stole furniture and electronics. Random shoot-outs broke out on the streets.

Sandro got a full taste of the new reality during his first day. He drove to Nino's apartment building and parked his car. Minutes later, when he looked out the windows of her apartment, he saw two strangers popping open the hood of his Zhiguli. By the time he ran out onto the street, they had stolen the battery. Sandro sprinted after the two men, who ran up to another building and shouted to their friend who was looking out the window, "We got it, Mito, we got it!" Just then, Sandro caught up, angry and ready for battle. "No, Mito, they ain't got it," he hollered at the man up high. "This is my battery, and I am taking it!" The duo didn't fight, so he carried the unit back to his car, but in the process, he splashed his new leather jacket with battery acid and ruined it. "The jacket probably cost me more than the new battery would," he recalls, but overall, he was lucky his robbers weren't armed.

Nino and Sandro got married, celebrating with a small circle of close friends—contrary to a typical Georgian wedding that often included upward of five hundred people drinking, singing, and dancing all night long. With the marriage certificate in hand, they applied for Nino's visa, and Sandro flew back home, now busy not only with *Yersinia* but also with living arrangements. The Morrises helped him find and furnish an apartment.

In May 1994, when Nino went to the recently established American consulate in Tbilisi, the counselor evaluating her visa application grew suspicious. She had just married a guy who himself had recently arrived in America—what was that about? Nino's answers about dating Sandro for a few years and his exciting research endeavors were to no avail. The counselor deemed their marriage fake and denied Nino's visa.[2]

Sandro was devastated. If he couldn't bring Nino, he didn't want to stay. Not only was he lonely, but he didn't want her to be left behind in a city where she could get hit by a stray bullet or a hijacked car. He spent several days in despair, staring into the distance rather than into his petri dishes. He needed to do more *Yersinia* experiments, but he was too depressed to focus on his work. He started talking about going back home. Seeing his postdoc in this miserable state, Morris began writing letters.

He wrote to the US ambassador in Tbilisi. He wrote to the US consul. He gathered signatures from the University of Maryland's officials. He praised Sandro as one of the brightest scientists he had ever known. "The work Dr. Sulakvelidze has done here has been outstanding so consequently we offered him a research position," he wrote. He assured the embassy bureaucrats that the marriage was not fake and that Sandro and Nino had been together for several years—and were very much in love. "As to the legitimacy of their marriage, Dr. Sulakvelidze has been talking about Nino ever since he arrived, and his stay was contingent upon her being able to join him," Morris stated. He wrote how excited Sandro was about finally reuniting with his now wife. "I have helped him find a new apartment here in Baltimore in preparation for her arrival and buy furniture."[3]

Finally, he wrote about how depressed and dejected Sandro had been since Nino's visa denial—so miserable, in fact, that he hadn't been able to do any work. "I can also tell you that he has spent the last two days moping around the laboratory worried about her; if we can't get this resolved I will lose a topflight fellow." The counselor's decision was unreasonable, he insisted. "According to the director of our university visa office this is the first time in 20 years that she has ever heard of her valid request for a J2 visa being declined."[4] He mailed the letters to every name he could find—and waited.

On the other side of the globe, Nino received an unexpected phone call. A clerk from the US embassy invited her to come back—not on the day when the consulate typically interviewed visa applicants but when the office was in fact closed. Nino was let into a quiet, empty building, where a consul ushered her into his office and issued her a visa to the United States. Glenn's letters did their magic—and now Sandro could go back to scrutinizing *Yersinia*. Nino was on her way.

The next step in Sandro's American life was buying a car—a scene Morris still remembers vividly thirty years later. "He showed up in a purple Chevrolet Camaro—a brightly colored model that dealers keep in the showrooms to attract people," Morris recalls with a smile. "He said, 'I dreamed of having something like this my entire life. And now I have it.' For him, it was part of becoming an American, and my wife and I thoroughly enjoyed helping both of them settle here."[5]

Nino was equally fascinated by America. Every day when Sandro left for work, she would go for a walk around Baltimore, admiring the neat houses, the beckoning shops, the splendid harbor. It was the antithesis to her chaotic homeland. "I was so amazed of how many opportunities were here," she recalls. "And how different everything was, even basic things. It was like learning to live all over again."

One of the most dramatic differences was having a baby in America. "In Georgia, I would've been drinking with friends, waiting for somebody to come and give me the news," Sandro recalls, since traditionally fathers were not permitted in the delivery room. "But here I was delivering the baby!" When he brought his son home, he immediately mailed the first batch of pictures to his father, Levan. With the way things were going, his dad wouldn't have the chance to hold his grandson for a while, so the pictures were the next best thing.

Levan did not live to receive them.

The envelope took several weeks to reach Tbilisi, and a heart attack killed Levan before the end of the month. Sandro left Nino alone with the baby—named Levan in the memory of the grandfather he'd never know—and flew home to bury his father. Glenn and Deborah Morris took care of Nino and little Levan in his absence. "They were regularly coming to check on me, they were bringing food, they were asking what I needed," she recalls. "They took care of us like we were family."

It was some months later that Morris lost his patient to

vancomycin-resistant enterococcus (VRE) and showed up in his lab with a forlorn look on his face, prompting Sandro to ask his phage question. The country with some of the highest standards of living and nearly limitless opportunities lacked the basic medicines Sandro's family had relied on his whole life. He couldn't wrap his mind around it. He couldn't understand why no one here ever heard of the concept.

"There was really no scientific literature on phages available in English," Morris says, reflecting on his first introduction to living medicines. "Most of the literature was in Russian, and I don't read Russian. All I could find in English was that this therapy had been tried earlier in the United States, and it fell out of favor. So it was really Sandro who educated me on what phages were and what their potential was." Morris didn't want to lose any more patients to VRE, so he listened. Like any practicing physician, he was always interested in what works. If phages worked in Georgia, they would work in America.

No average American clinician in the United States would try phages for treating bacterial infections. But as a physician who was also a researcher, Morris was in a more favorable position. He had a lab. He had research staff. He could submit proposals for funding. "As a scientist, I can test ideas," he says—no matter how crazy they sound. "So I said, let's write a couple of grant proposals and see what happens."[6]

The duo put together a proposal with an outlined scope of work and submitted it for grant applications. "We had no experience with FDA approvals and pharmaceutical manufacturing," says Sandro, but they had to start somewhere. Neither did they know anything about Good Manufacturing Practice (GMP) standards—a set of stringent FDA-established regulations, which ensure that pharmaceutical products are safe, pure, effective, and traceable. These rules dictate how the ingredients must be sourced. They require labeling and recordkeeping so everything can be traced—and, in case of a problem, recalled. The rules also outline sanitation conditions, which go far beyond merely keeping the production rooms sterilized. One of the requirements is keeping the facility at a higher pressure than the surrounding areas, to prevent any microorganisms from entering from the outside. Sandro and Morris were hoping to figure this out on the go. "We felt we knew what we had to do from the scientific standpoint," Morris says. "And we were hoping to find somebody who knew the rest of it."

Securing money even for basic phage research proved much easier said than done. The concept of using viruses to fight bacteria was so foreign that no agencies would entertain the idea. "People were looking at us like we were crazies," Sandro says. "They said, 'Forget about it. Don't even think about funding. You will never get money for something so ridiculous.' Even when I told them that I grew up using phages as medicines, they would laugh at me."

That was the situation when Sandro got a call from Nina Chanishvili. "We have an American businessman who wants to start a phage research company with our institute," Chanishvili told him over the phone. "Are you interested?"

ALL ROADS LEAD TO TBILISI

Sandro sat at his office at the University of Maryland School of Medicine, waiting for Caisey Harlingten to show up. "I was expecting an 'American businessman,' a man wearing a suit and tie," he says—an image he pictured in his head based on Chanishvili's description. "And there comes this guy dressed in jeans, sneakers, and a leather jacket." Harlingten said he had lost his luggage, but Sandro didn't necessarily believe it. "I have used that excuse a couple of times myself," he chuckles. Regardless, he liked the guy.

Only a few years older than Sandro, Harlingten had a gentle voice and mild manners, and he was keen on the idea of testing phages against the VRE. "He seemed genuinely interested in doing business with the Eliava Institute," Sandro says.

The VRE proposal that Sandro and Glenn had put together was finally useful. "Caisey signed a small contract with the University of Maryland," Sandro says. The next step was to test whether any of Eliava's phages were indeed effective against the Maryland VRE.

Sandro and Glenn gathered five hundred VRE samples collected from Maryland patients and mailed them to Tbilisi. Stuck inside glass vials with tight yellow lids, the samples were packaged in containers labeled INFECTIOUS SUBSTANCE and addressed to Nina Chanishvili, who by then had already set up a small lab with Harlingten's money. Overlooking the lush greenery of the Eliava campus, the lab had neat rows of tables, big windows that let in ample light, and equipment necessary to do the work. Equally important was the fact that the lab had continuously running water and steady electricity—a luxury many other labs didn't have.[7]

When the box arrived, the technicians set to work. They seeded petri dishes with the VRE samples, which, to a naked eye, looked like white stripes painted on the glass, each with an assigned number. Then the women dropped tiny quantities of phages from the Eliava collection into the stripes, hoping that some of them would prove to be good destroyers. Clad in white lab coats and black summer sandals, they walked down to the outfall of sewage pipes at the Mtkvari River, just like d'Hérelle and Eliava had done decades before. Standing at the observation deck above, they tied a glass lab bottle to a cotton rope and dangled it underneath the spitting brown stream until it was about half-full. They pulled it up, closed it tight, and carried it back to the lab. If no existing phages in the Eliava collection destroyed the VRE, those fished from sewage would surely do the job.

In the lab, the technicians held the petri dishes up to the light, looking for the telltale empty spots where the phages had chewed through bacterial colonies. Manually matching five hundred bacterial samples to phages took time, but their effort bore fruit. One day, the stripe marked *19* showed the unmistakable *taches vierges* that d'Hérelle described in his first "invisible microbe" paper back in 1917. Soon, a few other white stripes showed even larger empty spots. The white bands of VRE bacteria had been slashed, now looking patchy and uneven. "You could clearly see how the antibiotic-resistant strains were killed by the phages," Chanishvili says. "So we had phages effective against their VRE, and we could start manufacturing them at any moment." Halfway across the world, Georgian bacteria eaters were ready to save lives in Baltimore.[8] If they were approved by the FDA, of course.

Delighted with this first success, Harlingten organized a phage conference in a Communist-era retreat up in the mountains above Tbilisi. The event drew scientists from across the United States and Europe. Some of them did basic science research, some had used phages to treat livestock, while others had used phages to save humans. The researchers were beyond excited—some of them had spent their careers trying to convince policymakers to use phages as mainstream medicine, to no avail. Some had been laughed at by their colleagues. Now, someone was finally listening. And not just listening but taking important notes. The news reached the BBC, who sent a film crew to work on a documentary about the forgotten cure.

The BBC filmed the preparation of VRE samples in Baltimore and the phage production in Tbilisi. They interviewed Sandro and Glenn. They spoke to Nina and Teimuraz. At the conference, the BBC cameramen captured smiling people clinking champagne flutes, surrounded by mouthwatering desserts. They also filmed scientific reports and business discussions. "We will develop therapeutics together until we are ready to patent them," Teimuraz

Chanishvili told BBC about the imminent collaboration. "Then we will decide who and how will mass-produce the preparations."[9]

Everything looked promising, but trouble already was compromising the partnership.

Harlingten brought with him his CEO, Richard Honour, whose job was to figure out how to make the phage collaboration work to satisfy the stringent FDA approval requirements. Honour had the right qualifications and the track record. He spent a decade running a massive cancer clinical trials research program at the University of Southern California in Los Angeles, where he worked on getting drugs approved by the FDA on a daily basis. "We had hundreds of affiliated institutions all over the US and Canada, we had thousands of doctors, full-time staff of 43 clinical analysts and seven biostatisticians," Honour recalls. He knew exactly what the FDA would want and how hard it would be to pass all the agency's milestones. And he was very vocal about it, every step of the way.[10]

He didn't think the nascent Georgia Research Institute could convince the FDA to manufacture phage therapeutics in a struggling former Soviet republic. He didn't think the Eliava Institute, which couldn't get the electricity to run reliably, could build a facility that was compliant with the stringent GMP practices. The bullet pockmarks scattered on buildings worried him as a sign of instability. For Harlingten, the dilapidated Eliava labs signaled an opportunity to revive its old glory and make money. For Honour, it was the reason to take business somewhere else.[11] "It was almost as if Caisey was playing a good cop and Richard was playing a bad cop," Sandro recalls. "And Richard was very forthcoming with his opinions."

"Nearly everyone in Tbilisi didn't like me within about 10 minutes of showing up," says Honour, who, at eighty-three years old, still remembers the trip as if it was yesterday. "But that's what I was brought there for. I was saying, of course, anything can be done if you have enough money. In this case, you have to build a complete infrastructure, but the US Food and Drug Administration is not going to smile favorably on such a facility in Georgia, unless you really can bring it up to Western standards."[12]

At one point in the conference, Honour drew a map of what it would take to get the FDA's greenlight. The lecture became known as "the rock talk," he says, because he sketched it out on a massive slab of black slate that was somehow brought into the auditorium in lieu of a missing blackboard. "There wasn't any chalk or anything to write with, so I walked out into the yard outside the university and found a piece of white cement that had been blown off a building. And I used that piece of white cement as white chalk for my chalk," Honour recalls. "I wrote on this giant black slate board the basic outline of the FDA regulatory process for the development and approval of a new antimicrobial agent. The slate was about twenty-five feet by five or six feet, and I wrote on it from left to right. And then I went along the drawing, and I pointed out all the shortcomings. I was trying to be very objective and honest, and the audience just got more and more furious with me." Honour maintains that he wasn't unsympathetic, just realistic. "Tbilisians really wanted to have a good professional outcome from their hundred years' worth of work on phages. But from my experience I knew it was going to be very difficult to pull off."[13]

By the time the conference ended, Harlingten was convinced he wouldn't be able to organize the phage production in Tbilisi. So instead, he decided to set up a phage center in Seattle.[14] When Honour and Harlingten went back home, they offered a contract that asked for exclusive access to the institute's knowledge, but for a fraction of the cost that was discussed. The institute refused to accept the terms, and the discussions broke down.

Shortly after, Harlingten wrote to Sandro that he still wanted to work with him and Glenn. And at the same time, Honour showed the BBC a new phage production facility they began building near Seattle.[15] "All of that didn't feel right to us," Sandro says. "We started this project with Nina and the Eliava Institute, and then they just got cut off." Glenn and Sandro were hesitant to work with partners who changed directions so drastically. Ultimately, the two chose to part ways with Harlingten and Honour but keep their ties with the Eliava Institute. "There came a point where we realized that what made the most sense was creating a small company," Morris says. "And then get some phage products here from Georgia and work toward the FDA approvals."

Sandro wrote Nina an email, explaining that they decided to form their own venture. She took the news bitterly. To her, this was a loss of the opportunity and investment necessary to revive the Eliava Institute and the livelihoods of her colleagues—a lifeline. She also saw it as a betrayal of her trust. "I was the one who connected them with Harlingten," she says, still disappointed, years later. "And instead, he decided to create his own company. That's not what I asked him for."

Sandro and Glenn saw the move as the necessary path forward. With a company of their own, they hoped to work with the FDA on setting up the required tests, documenting the process and the outcomes, and eventually securing the agency's approval. "Although once we got into it, we realized that it would be a lot more complicated than we imagined," Glenn admits. "But forming a company was a start."[16]

LYSIS TO KILL

"You're looking for a hundred thousand dollars to prove that these phages can destroy antibiotic-resistant bacteria?" John Woloszyn, a partner at McGuireWoods, a US-based international law firm, was not at all swayed by the amount. "I can write you a check for that today."[17]

Sandro and Morris were sitting at Woloszyn's corner office in the McGuireWoods building that overlooked downtown Baltimore through beautiful windows. Morris's neighbor, who was friends with Woloszyn, had organized the meeting because the two scientists needed a lawyer to get them incorporated. Now, it seemed that they had more than legal counsel. They had found their first investor. "Woloszyn's take on the whole phage endeavor was 'Why are you wasting time with all those people?'" Sandro recalls. "'You need a few bucks to start? Let's move ahead.'"

Intralytix was born in June 1998, its name inspired by the word *lytic*, which came from phages lysing their host. Sandro had a good feeling about the new venture.

If only he knew how far from his goal he really was.

He had no idea of the approval hurdles that loomed ahead. Many of them stemmed from the fact that inconsistent phage preparations had all but discredited the treatment in the early twentieth century. A number of scientists were skeptical of so-called commie remedies. And living medicines didn't fit neatly into the FDA's approval pathway. The chief regulatory obstacle was that phages—like any viruses, bacteria, and organisms in general—change constantly. Unlike the set molecules of traditional medicines—antibiotics, fever reducers, painkillers, and glucose stabilizers—phages evolve from one generation to the next. They don't change drastically, but they tweak their genomes by altering a few genes here and there. Moreover, they multiply inside the patients. How does one decide how much phage to give?

That presented a tough conundrum for the FDA because—for the most part—the agency's traditional duty had been assuring that manufactured medicines *don't change.*

Traditional medicines don't alter their molecular formula or structure from one batch to the next. The active ingredients in amoxicillin and ciprofloxacin are defined, quantified, and clinically tested to receive the coveted FDA-approval stamp. Any significant deviation in their chemical composition must go through the rigorous and expensive testing processes to get the same stamp again, after which the new compound might even receive a different name. The approved manufacturing process is followed exactly— inside the state-of-the-art GMP facilities where every vial is labeled and traceable—which guarantees the same results, always.

Phages are different. They aren't synthesized chemically. They assemble themselves inside a bacterial organism. As they do that, they can drop a gene. Or they can pick up a few new ones. The progeny won't be drastically dissimilar, but they will differ just enough to present a problem—they are no longer the same. Does it mean that the new phage or phage cocktail must go through clinical trials again? And what if you needed to mutate an existing phage because the bacteria it preys on has mutated and developed a resistance? That's why Eliava Institute scientists collected germs from all over the USSR and constantly developed new phages to keep up with the bugs, but—for better or for worse—they didn't put the new formulations through rigorous clinical trials every time they added a new bacteria eater in the mix.

All that made it very difficult for phages to earn FDA approval. The agency has two different departments for evaluating therapeutics. One is called the Center for Drug Evaluation and Research, or CDER, which evaluates medicines that are chemically synthesized—such as antibiotics. The other is the Center for Biologics Evaluation and Research, or CBER, which regulates products derived from living sources, whether humans, animals, or microorganisms—such as flu vaccines, which may change from one season to the next. As biological entities, phages would fall under CBER regulations, but they still differed from many other medicines the department regulated and remained a fairly foreign, puzzling, and untrustworthy entity.

There are many important reasons for the FDA's strict scrutiny. That seemingly rigid approval approach is crucial for producing the unparalleled accuracy of our medicines. That oversight guarantees that our amoxicillin or doxycycline destroy bacteria the same way in every person who takes them. The rigorous testing assures that our biologics work as expected, every time. That repeatability and reproducibility is what made the mass production of medicines so successful in public health.

That is also what made us a victim of our own success. In our quest for that reliably repeatable sameness of our medicinal molecules, we forgot that germs evolve while the drugs don't. These inanimate compounds can't play catch-up with bacterial defenses. The very VRE that Sandro and Glenn wanted to treat with phages was a perfect example of that problem. In April 2000—after years in development—the FDA approved an antibiotic called *linezolid* to treat the VRE. Less than a year later, a new VRE strain was already resistant. The bug took less time to evolve its defenses than we took to develop ours.[18]

"When particular bacteria develop an antibiotic resistance, it takes several years and several million dollars to develop a new antibiotic," Sandro says. "And by the time the new drug is approved or shortly after doctors start using it, the mutant strains resistant to it start to appear, so we are back to square one."

That day, when he became the CEO of Intralytix, Sandro had no idea how many times he would find himself back to that very same square.

11

The Phage Whisperer

Biswajit Biswas drew a syringe full of phage and injected it into his laboratory mice, one after another. The mice weren't sick, so he wasn't using phages as medicine. He just wanted to know how long the phages would persist inside the mice—an experiment similar to what Eliava and d'Hérelle once carried out to understand how far phages could travel in rodents' bodies. In about a day, Biswas would test the mice's blood to see if the phages were still floating inside them. Typically, most phages would be gone because they were quickly filtered by the liver and spleen, but sometimes a tiny fraction remained. Biswas would harvest the survivors, grow them—and inject them into the mice again.

Biswas was working on this unconventional project in the mid-1990s, in the laboratory of Carl Merril, an NIH scientist and an early phage enthusiast who was playing around with the idea of using them to treat disease. Their mice were getting blood tests right about the same time that Sandro and Morris were having their first phage conversations and putting together their VRE proposals. Geographically, the two teams weren't far from each other. Both were located in Maryland. Both understood phages as medicinal agents, which the rest of the medical field viewed as nonsensical.[1]

Merril, however, approached the problem from a different angle. Rather than treating sick mice with phages, he wanted to know how long living medicines could survive inside a creature. In humans and animals, the liver, spleen, and immune system tackle foreign invaders and filter them out quickly. Merril wanted to know how long phages could persist before they got gobbled up by the body's natural defense mechanisms. He also wanted to know if phages could evolve to avoid being devoured. By hand-picking surviving phages and reinjecting them again, Biswas and Merril hoped to find answers.

"It was a selection process," Biswas explains. "I was growing phages and injecting them intravenously and intraperitoneally in mice, and the next day, after thirteen or eighteen hours, I would bleed the mice and take those phages and grow it again—passage after passage." It was a method akin to what d'Hérelle outlined in his book *The Bacteriophage and the Phenomenon of Recovery*, which Eliava translated.[2]

Originally from India, Biswas followed his family's tradition and earned a degree in veterinary medicine. Working in animal husbandry in the mid-1980s, he watched with growing concern the increasing use of antibiotics—both to battle infections and to fatten up the animals. While looking for possible alternatives, he came across intriguing scientific literature dating back to the early twentieth century, when d'Hérelle's successful phage experiments prompted doctors to first use them to treat disease.[3] Between 1930 and 1935, British medical officer Lieutenant Colonel J. Morison, who was inspired by d'Hérelle's work, used phages during cholera epidemics in India, for treatment and prevention.[4] In 1932, he reported few cholera deaths in the phage-treated Naogaon region, compared to 474 deaths in the Habiganj region that declined to utilize the treatment.[5] "I read a paper that the British actually used bacteriophage from River Ganges to treat cholera," says Biswas. "They inoculated a water well in a village, and that reduced the incidences of cholera."[6]

As a veterinarian in India, Biswas didn't have a way to experiment with phages. But then, like Sandro, he came to the United

States in the 1990s to work on his PhD. He landed in the same place as Sandro, the University of Maryland. There, he found an ally in Merril, who was equally fascinated with bacteria eaters. As an NIH scientist, Merril watched antibiotics lose their punch and knew medicine needed an alternative. "When I started my career in the 1970s, we thought antibiotics were doing fine. By the 1990s, it was clear that we were going to have a problem. I thought phages were worth trying."[7]

Merril had become interested in bacteriophages after taking a summer course at Cold Spring Harbor back in the 1970s. The course focused on phages' basic biology, but for Merril, it left two big unanswered questions.[8]

"Why don't we use them for treating infectious diseases?" Merril asked his professor. The man told him to go read *Arrowsmith* by Sinclair Lewis—the very book that left d'Hérelle excited in the spring of 1925, shortly before he so spectacularly cured plague in Egypt. The professor's intention was to show Merril why phages had become discredited, but that wasn't what he found. In fact, Merril realized that his professor likely skimmed the book, if he read it at all. "He didn't read *Arrowsmith*, because if you read it really carefully, it's not an indictment of phage," Merril says. "It's an indictment of human beings and their greed and their misuse of things."[9]

Merril's other big question was about what happens to phages once they enter the human body—in particular, the circulatory system. Does the immune system destroy them? How quickly? Can some persist? From initial experiments with injecting phages into mice, he found that even before the immune system cells gobbled up bacteriophages as foreign organisms, the liver and spleen filtered them out. "My next question was, can we find a phage strain that wouldn't be taken up by the liver?" he recalls. "Such a strain would be more effective."

Merril happened to be on a committee that oversaw Biswas's PhD research, and one day, they started talking. "I told him that I used phages before in my graduate studies to make a phage library mainly for molecular biology work," Biswas recalls. Merril was interested. "I'd like to try to use bacteriophages to overcome antibiotic resistance problems," he told Biswas. "Would you come work in my lab?"[10] Biswas was intrigued. "I said, 'It's an interesting idea. I can work in that field.'"[11]

For a while after he joined Merril's lab, Biswas's days revolved around injecting mice with phages against *E.coli* and *Salmonella typhimurium* and then taking their blood tests to see how quickly the bacteria eaters were eaten themselves, disappearing from circulation. About a day later, most phages would be gone, except for a tiny fraction. Biswas would filter them—and repeat the process again. The first few rounds didn't exhibit much success. But then Biswas noticed that the survivors' numbers increased. "Surprisingly, after the eleventh round, we saw that the phage titer from the blood was getting higher," he recalls. "So we isolated those long-circulating or long-swimming phages." Similarly to d'Hérelle, they also turned to Greek mythology, naming their newfound potent creatures after Jason and the Argonauts, who sailed on the ship called *Argo* to retrieve the Golden Fleece. Although technically speaking phages can't swim on their own, they merely float, Biswajit and Merril liked the term. "We called them Argo1 and Argo2 phages because they were good swimmers."[12]

The two types of Argo phages Biswas and Merril selected weren't just good swimmers—they were exceptional. Argo1's eighteen-hour survival numbers were sixteen-thousand-fold higher than the strain Biswas started with. Argo2's was thirteen-thousand-fold higher. Notably, these Argo phages also made better medicines than their original brethren. "Mice would survive when you treat with either phage," Biswas says. "But when we treated them with the Argo phages, they would recover much faster because the phages persisted longer in their bodies."[13]

Eventually, Merril and Biswas sequenced the Argos and zeroed in on exactly what made them "good swimmers," capable of avoiding the entrapment of mice livers and spleens. "It was a tiny mutation in one gene, caused by a change in one amino acid, that resulted in a change on the phage's surface," Biswas says." The finding was so bizarre that another scientist set off to double-check it by specifically mutating the implicated gene—and proved it true. "The single-point mutation kept the phage in the circulation of a mouse more than ten-thousand-fold longer," Merril says, still in awe of Mother Nature's tricks. It was evolution's spectacular handiwork. "That showed that phages are also adapting and are trying to survive," Biswas says, "because they don't want to be grabbed by the liver and get destroyed."[14]

When Biswas and Merril published their paper in 1996, setting forth the idea of revisiting phages as medicinal agents, the scientific world was not amused. Similar to Sandro and Morris's experience, Biswas and Merril's ideas were dismissed. In the 1990s doctrine, phages belonged in the lab and not in the clinic. A committee evaluating Merril's proposal to advance phage therapeutics was not amused either. His argument about using phage to combat antibiotic resistance didn't resonate at all. "The committee said, 'This is ridiculous. Eventually, the bacteria will become resistant to the phage,'" Merril recalls with frustration. "Moreover, they said, 'The resistance will occur very quickly. So we're not going to let you do that.' Of course, in the meantime, we could have saved all those patients, but that's irrelevant."[15]

Just like D'Hérelle, who lost his lab space to Pasteur Institute politics, Merril's funding was drastically cut due to his unconventional experiments. The Pasteur scientists made fun of d'Hérelle chasing the "invisible microbes," and Merril's NIH colleagues ridiculed his obsession with viruses that could cure. But just like d'Hérelle, he was too driven to give up.

Instead, he founded a spin-off company, Exponential Biotherapies, which aimed to develop bacteriophages for a slew of antibiotic-resistant infections ranging from MRSA to VRE, to multidrug-resistant pseudomonas, *E. coli*, campylobacter, and listeria. He brought Biswas along too. Once again, the team had very similar goals to what Sandro and Morris set off to do with Intralytix—convince the FDA that phages were safe and efficient antibiotic alternatives. They began with mice and were hoping to move on to human trials.

In 2002, Merril, Biswas, and their coworkers published a paper demonstrating a near-miraculous VRE phage result on mice. Mice infected with VRE strains recently collected from patients died within two days. When treated with phages shortly after infection, all of them recovered. If researchers waited with treatments until the animals were so sick they were nearly dying, half of them still bounced back after a single injection. "With the emergence of antibiotic-resistant bacteria, such as VRE and methicillin-resistant Staphylococcus aureus, there is a need to explore the potential therapeutic applications of bacteriophages," the authors wrote. The paper, however, stirred up little enthusiasm in the larger scientific community.

The following year, Merril, along with collaborators Dean Scholl and Sankar L. Adhya, wrote another paper titled "The Prospect for Bacteriophage Therapy in Western Medicine" and published it in the journal *Nature*. In the paper, Merril sounded the alarm, pointing out that 70 percent of hospital-acquired bacterial infections in the United States were now resistant to one or more of the main antibiotics. Then, once again, he described phages as the alternatives. He dug into history, telling the stories of d'Hérelle's treatment triumphs. He noted that phages were successfully used in the US in the 1930s. He even told the brief story of the Eliava Institute, noting its phage production throughout the Soviet era and World War II. He then went on to examine a vast assemblage of literature about phage therapy, pointing out its potential, its existing flaws, and its future opportunities. He cited cases where phages were successfully used to treat antibiotic-resistant infections in mice, including VRE and MRSA.[16]

Merril's answer to the previous committee's concern about bacteria becoming phage-resistant was to develop a library of phages, keeping track of which phage killed what bug. He also envisioned using not one single phage but a phage cocktail so that if patients were infected by multiple bacterial variants or if bacteria mutated inside them, the "phage team" would kill it anyway. "I took it to heart what they said about bacteria becoming resistant," he says. His vision was very similar to what the Soviet Ministry of Health implemented in 1967, when it began collecting pathogenic bacteria from across the country and sending the bacteria to the Eliava Institute to breed phages that killed them. The Soviets had gathered over forty-two thousand bacteria strains, but the number of phages that dwell on earth is much greater. "We estimate that the number of phages on this planet is ten to the power of thirty-one," Merril says. "There are so many phages in the world that you don't have to worry about bacteria developing resistance to them all. We'll never run out of them."[17]

The American scientific community wasn't persuaded by these ideas either, so in 2005, another committee recommended to close Merril's lab—another uncanny similarity to d'Hérelle's path. Merril was nearing retirement, so he did just that. He had a big house, a garden to tend, and a slew of hobbies to indulge in. His son, Greg, was competing at car races and Merril often traveled with him, so he had plenty to do.[18]

Biswas, on the contrary, still needed a job, so he bounced between different start-ups, always keeping his focus on phages. He lived and breathed phages, sometimes quite literally. As fate would have it, his house was down the road from a sewage treatment plant, so close that he could see it driving to work. On hot summer days, the seething muck would begin to smell, and Biswas reveled in the stink. "Oh, what a perfect day to hunt for phages," he would tell his wife—and then he would call the plant for permission to come and collect the stinky water. "When it smells really bad, I know there's more phage and they are thriving," he explains. The spiking temperatures make bacteria proliferate faster than usual. As they grow, they release noxious gases, such as hydrogen sulfide, which smells like rotten eggs or rotten shoes, Biswas says. "And anything that smells rotten means that bacteria are growing. And the more they're growing, the more phage grows too. The smellier it is, the more diverse phages we will get."

Among his colleagues, Biswas became known as a phage whisperer, a person who intuitively knew where to look for the right phage and how to pit it against the right bacteria. Yet despite his rare talents, holding on to a job that involved phages proved difficult. For a while, Biswas was developing phage-based vaccines at Hygea BioPharma. The idea was to use a phage to deliver a snippet of a pathogen into an organism so that the immune system would learn to recognize it—just like Covid vaccines introduced a piece of the spike protein to draw the immune system's response. Eventually, Hygea folded. After that, Biswas went to Panacea Pharmaceuticals, where he developed various bacteriophages for therapeutic and prophylactic uses. Panacea Pharmaceuticals didn't last either. None of the phage start-ups lasted long. The viruses were unpopular subjects.

At some point, Sandro and Biswas crossed paths. Biswas was looking for a job, and Intralytix was pursuing a new research project. "We talked about various projects," Biswas says. "He's a renowned phage scientist and he used to work at the Baltimore campus of the University of Maryland. He worked very hard to get phages off the ground, and he kept hitting the wall. But we never collaborated." Biswas wanted to study phages for therapeutic purposes, and Intralytix didn't have the funds for medical research and was forced to focus on other applications to make money. So Biswas continued looking for work, and Sandro continued looking for investors.

The world just wasn't interested in phage whisperers. At least, not yet.

12

Naive and Stubborn,
a Winning Combination

The truckloads full of fresh fish began to arrive at Inverness—a city in the Scottish Highlands—in early morning. The workers at Strathaird Salmon, the company that turned the catch into delectable smoked fillets, off-loaded the cargo, taking it into the processing docks. As always, they washed, cleaned, and sliced the fish, but this time—on a cold and gloomy Monday morning in January 2008—they added an extra step at the end. They let the visiting crew of three Intralytix employees treat the sea's bounty with ListShield—a phage that kills *Listeria monocytogenes*, a common pathogen that contaminates food, including salmon. The crew, which included Sandro, his then CEO John Vazzana, and a technician, sprayed the salmon samples with the invisible bacteria destroyers. Once they were done, they kept half the samples in-house and sent the other half to a third-party company to conduct an independent test of ListShield efficacy against *L. monocytogenes*. And then they waited.

Twenty-five million dollars was at stake.

A prominent US company was interested in buying Strathaird to bring the pink delicacy to the American consumers. That market was huge, but there was a catch. American seafood regulations had zero tolerance for listeria while Scottish ones were more relaxed. To get Scottish fish into American supermarkets, it had to be guaranteed listeria-free. The company hired Intralytix to do the test and promised to invest the $25 million if it worked. This was the biggest opportunity Sandro's venture had encountered since its inception.[1]

On the eve of its tenth anniversary, Intralytix still had not made a big breakthrough, persevering despite a number of setbacks and a steady drum of naysayers, certain that no phage ideas would ever succeed in the US. But Sandro was undeterred. He had never been good at giving up. And he wouldn't give up now.

Shortly after forming Intralytix, Sandro set up a phage lab at the University of Maryland and brought over a Georgian crew from Tbilisi. Headed by Zemphira Alavidze, who had once led the Eliava Institute's Laboratory of Morphology and Biology of Phages, the crew was teaching their American colleagues phage wisdom dating back to d'Hérelle's 1930s monograph: how to hunt for bacterial eaters in local sewage, how to grow them in large numbers, how to purify and make efficient phage preparations. Once they had enough data, Sandro and Morris put together a proposal about using phages to treat the old nemesis—the vancomycin-resistant enterococcus—and sent it to the NIH and the FDA.

On a fateful day in June 2001, Sandro, full of hope and ambitions, drove in his purple Camaro to a meeting with both agencies. The former was open to his idea, the latter not so much.[2]

One of the FDA's concerns was that not all phages are created equal. At the basic level, phages split into two distinct camps: the lytic and the lysogenic. The lytic phages are the ones that lyse the bacteria—burst, pierce, and destroy it. The lysogenic ones are trickier. They don't destroy when they infect. Instead, they insert their DNA into the genome of their host, and when the bacteria replicate, the phage replicates with it. Needless to say, such phages are useless for therapy. Because of their "mild temperament," they are sometimes called the *temperate phages,* or at least so the saying goes. But the name is a misnomer, because temperate phages can, in a roundabout way, be quite dangerous—not to the bacteria but to humans.

Sometimes when these lysogenic phages wiggle into their host's genome, that extra DNA snippet can make the bacteria function differently—for example, release a toxin. That toxin can make the originally harmless germ far more pathogenic. One such temperate phage may have caused the great throat distemper of 1735, which killed a third of all children in New England, according to Carl Merril. It may have invaded a relatively benign bacteria *Corynebacterium diphtheriae* and plugged itself into its DNA, which made the bacteria secrete a toxin that disrupts the production of vital proteins in humans—and caused the infamous diphtheria outbreaks.[3] In fact,[4] a temperate phage may have made *Vibrio cholerae* bacteria far more deadly than it had once been.[5]

Lysogenic phages are unreliable and dangerous—if not as much for a specific patient but on a global scale because they can turn relatively mild bugs into brutal killers. When making therapeutic cocktails, scientists want to deal with lytic ones only—the proven assassins that don't cause any genetic mutations. This level of phage finesse wasn't possible during d'Hérelle and Eliava's era but became achievable with modern electron microscopy and genome-sequencing techniques. Yet, the FDA didn't think that Sandro's plan had convincingly demonstrated that his therapeutic cocktails would contain lytic phages only and assure that no temperate ones could sneak in.

Sandro agreed that this concern was legitimate, and he could implement more checks in his production techniques. Other requests he found unrealistic. "The FDA asked me to determine how quickly each of the six phages in the VRE cocktail would mutate

inside our mice and how these mutations will affect their microbiome," he recalls. "That wasn't possible to do in any reasonable
amount of time with any reasonable resources."

To Sandro, this gap stemmed from the lack of understanding
that phages were different from antibiotics, looping back to the
concept that medical formulas aren't expected to change. "I could
see that you can spend five or ten years analyzing a formula and
then you would use it for the next thirty," he says. "But phages don't
work like that. They may need to be remixed every few years."[6]

He also disagreed that such a fine level of scrutiny made any
sense. "I think the issue of temperate versus lytic is a little overblown," he says. "Of course, I would use lytic phages rather than
temperate because, for starters, they do their job much better—
invade bacteria, multiply and kill it, while temperate ones don't.
Safety wise, I am not sure this is really that critical. For example, the
human gastrointestinal tract naturally has about ten to the power of
fifteen phages in it. Presumably at least half of them are temperate.
Who controls what they do in there?"[7]

He felt that while the agency's representatives didn't explicitly
turn his idea down, they essentially made it impossible to implement. He also wondered if phages were tainted by their very origin.
They came from the Soviet Union, a country that for decades was
locked in a Cold War standoff with America. How could this therapy be trusted?

Sandro was hoping to get grant money from the NIH to test
out his first phage cocktails in mice and gather as much data as
possible. One of his NIH contacts, the antimicrobial resistance
program officer Marissa Miller, encouraged Sandro and Morris to
give it a try. But getting funding for phage research proved impossible. Even when the agency received $20 million dollars from the
US Congress to develop new drugs to fight antibiotic resistance,
Sandro and Glenn didn't get a penny. "NIH came up with a chal-

lenge grant opportunity, so we applied," Sandro says. "And boy, did we get trashed!"[8]

Not only did they not receive any funding, but some naysayers published scathing letters in scientific journals condemning the idea because, they said, it had never worked. One paper published in *Nature* stated that "bacteriophage therapy for bacterial infections has almost a cult-like following," while there is no data on their efficiency, save for anecdotal and not credible evidence.[9] Some of the correspondence triggered a response from William Summers—the Yale University microbiologist and d'Hérelle's biographer—who wrote that phages, in fact, did work, and had been working for decades in other countries. Summers's response prompted another letter from the opposition.

"It was amazing to what extent some people were really against it," Sandro reflects. "We tried multiple times to get funding. I would write several grant applications. Glenn would write several grant applications. And we would get nowhere, despite the fact that Glenn is a supremely successful scientist who had received many NIH grants. The concept of phages as therapeutics was just too out of the box." American medicine wasn't interested in treating people with viruses, even the good ones.

The early 2000s were universally bad for phage research. In 2005, the Eliava Institute almost went out of existence because it couldn't make enough money to pay the bills. The Georgian government viewed it as a problem and wanted to merge it with other research institutions, which likely would have resulted in a massive loss of phage expertise. The institute survived only because the international scientific community stepped in to save its independence. "We also wrote a letter of support of the institute as an independent entity," Sandro says. The Georgian government listened. The scientists won. The Eliava Institute remained an independent entity.

Winning over the American scientific community was much harder. American scientists didn't drink living medicines when they were kids. "But I did!" Sandro points out. "I have seen it work. I grew up seeing it working. I knew phages would work again, so all I needed was to demonstrate it." For that, however, he needed money. And since the agencies weren't funding his ideas, he resolved to do it himself. "I had to figure out how to make my company profitable enough so I could use the money to do research and demonstrate the results."

Sandro changed course. He decided to introduce bacteria eaters from a different angle and a different regulatory process: food safety applications.

Getting a medicine approved takes series of lengthy and expensive clinical trials. But receiving approvals for food safety products takes significantly less time and money. So Sandro chose to focus on developing phages as antibacterial agents for poultry, meat, and produce. The Good Manufacturing Processes, or GMP, for the food industry are also much less rigorous and cheaper to achieve, so making phage sprays seemed like an easier target—and it could earn money quickly.

Every idea needs the right moment. In the early 2000s, the moment was right for phage food safety. At the time, many poultry and meat producers were beginning to curtail their antibiotic use. But they needed to keep their products bacteria-free. Achieving these two goals demanded an antibiotic alternative. One of the companies that took interest in Sandro's start-up was Perdue, one of America's largest poultry producers. Perdue was interested in efficient ways to keep their chicken breasts, thighs, and legs salmonella-free. The bug naturally dwells inside the birds' guts, rarely making them sick. However, when chickens are sliced and packaged, the germs inevitably end up contaminating at least some batches, where they grow and multiply. Some of those strains were already resistant to certain antibiotics, so Perdue was looking for alternatives.[10]

The company's microbiologists knew nothing about phages, but they were receptive to Sandro's vision. After several meetings and presentations, Perdue partnered with Intralytix and invested a million dollars into making phage sprays against salmonella and listeria.[11] "That was a big thing for us," Sandro recalls. "We could work on this alternative revenue stream, build the business, get a few products approved, find some distributors—and then try the medicine angle again."

Sandro's intuition was right. The phage spray approval took a few years, loads of data, and piles of documents, but it worked. In 2006, the FDA green-lighted Intralytix's inaugural invention: ListShield, a spray against *Listeria monocytogenes*, the first ever FDA-approved phage product for the food industry, and the first commercial phage preparation used in America since the 1930s. Sandro felt that his efforts finally broke the ice, or at least cracked it, when it came to winning over the FDA's attitude toward good viruses.

"At that time, Intralytix was the only company in the world—not just in America—to have received FDA approval for using a bacteriophage-based preparation as a food additive," Sandro says. "There was much joy. We felt like pioneers. We popped the champagne."

The milestone didn't translate into immediate financial boon. "We got a lot of media attention," Sandro says, but sales were slow. Customers weren't familiar with phages, and the concept of using viruses for food safety was foreign to them. Consumers were ill prepared too. A comment one reader left after reading an article about Intralytix's breakthrough left Sandro in awe. "They are spraying viruses on my meat?" the comment read. "What if the viruses are going to eat some of my meat? I already pay too much for my

meat and now I am going to get even less of it." The reader deemed
the phage idea a clever marketing trick aimed to drive up the price
of food. Years later, Sandro still remembers that comment. "I realized that we really needed a strong education campaign to explain
the science to people."

The deal with Perdue bridged Intralytix to its first approval, but
it didn't last. The person who pioneered the phage work at Perdue left the company, and research ground to a halt. "We lost our
champion," Sandro says—and had to start looking for other partners. And that's where the Strathaird Salmon deal came in. With
the $25 million deal looming ahead, Intralytix was poised to take
off. And then, Sandro could dust off the VRE project again and
give it another shot. As long as ListShield worked.[12]

The test was supposed to last five days, and Sandro diligently
checked the samples every morning. "We could go home and just
wait for the test results there, but we didn't want to," he recalls. "It
was so much more fun to watch it ourselves." For the remainder of
the day, they didn't have much to do, so they went around town
eating Scottish food and drinking different scotches for five days.
Loch Ness was nearby, so they ventured out to its shores, looking
for the elusive monster, Nessie.

The five days passed, and the test results from the third-party
company came back. They were spectacular. "There was not a trace
of listeria in the sprayed samples," Sandro says. The fish that wasn't
sprayed was chock-full of listeria, but the phage-treated salmon
was squeaky clean. "It was one hundred percent clear, so there was
no doubt we were getting our twenty-five million dollars."

Ecstatic, they went to celebrate in the best restaurant in town.
More plans were made. To commemorate the moment of this
Scottish success, no doubt fueled by the outsize quantities of
scotch, they considered buying kilts—and wearing them at Intralytix when they got home. "We almost did it," Sandro says. "The

only reason we didn't was that I wasn't flying directly home. So we couldn't show up in kilts together, and John didn't want to do it alone. At the end, we didn't buy the kilts."

They didn't get the $25 million either.

The American buyer changed its mind about acquiring Strathaird Salmon. They paid Intralytix a $250,000 success fee, but that was a far cry from their original promise. Sandro was crushed.[13]

For the next decade, which seemed like an eternity, Intralytix would keep struggling. Yet it persevered. The quarter of a million dollars helped it move forward. More interested parties joined the bandwagon, including the US military, which helped fund the development of salmonella and shigella phage sprays. Thanks to these investments, the FDA approved more food sprays over the next several years. Having achieved these milestones, Intralytix began designing combination cocktails, composed of different phages that targeted multiple bacteria species. One included phages for *E. coli*, salmonella, and listeria, germs that commonly cause food poisoning. The second covered shigella and campylobacter. With every approval, Intralytix inched forward, but it was still too far from being able to fund its own research. Selling these sprays helped keep the company afloat, but what it needed was a big breakthrough with enough money to revive the antibiotic alternative idea—and Intralytix just didn't seem to get one. It was too ahead of its time.

Most people would've given up, but Sandro couldn't let go. "I think it was my naïveté that got us through," he says, reflecting on his years of perseverance. "That—and my stubbornness. Everyone was saying, 'Forget it, it will never work. The FDA would never approve that.' And I just couldn't understand why *not*? Because using phages made so much sense. I knew they worked. I had seen them work. They were still working back home in Tbilisi. How could I give up?"

It was working, slowly. In regulatory framework, there is a

concept of substances generally recognized as safe, or GRAS. By painstakingly gathering data from their food sprays, Intralytix was slowly pushing phages toward that GRAS designation—in the agricultural realm to start with. And that was a big foundational shift that would, one day, play out in medicine too. "At least, that's what I hoped for," Sandro says. "I had to have hope."[14]

And one day, the shift came. Ushered in by a deadly, drug-resistant bacteria, a perfect storm uncovered the phages from almost a century of obscurity.

13

The Superbug That Won the Oscar—and the FDA

Thomas Patterson had been on about fifteen different antibiotics, including the toughest ones American pharma ever created. His running list of antibacterial weaponry included meropenem, tigecycline, vancomycin, daptomycin, rifampin, colistin, azithromycin, teicoplanin, metronidazole, and imipenem.[1] None of them worked. The vicious bug that Tom, then a sixty-eight-year-old behavioral psychologist from San Diego, contracted while vacationing in Egypt was ravaging his insides. He had been in a coma for weeks and on the brink of death multiple times. In fact, if he were just another human, he would have been long dead already. But Tom wasn't just another human—he was a lucky one. He was married to an infectious disease epidemiologist, Steffanie Strathdee, once nicknamed "Pit Bull" for her indomitable will.

Tom's monthslong battle with the antibiotic-resistant blight began on the dream trip the couple took over Thanksgiving week in 2015. One day, they had a rare opportunity to explore the Red Pyramid in Dahshur, typically closed because of its proximity to a military base. The only way to see the pyramid was to crawl inside it, a feat Steffanie wasn't up for, but Tom was. "Don't breathe the air," a watchman cautioned as Tom crawled inside—the locals believed the tomb accumulated noxious gases. The warning may have been ominous. Whether Tom actually picked up the bug inside the cold, dusty, decay-smelling enclosure would forever remain a mystery, but he began feeling unwell a few hours later. He seemed better the next morning, and after touring the Luxor and Karnak temples, the couple had a romantic dinner, celebrating the anniversary of their first date fourteen years prior.

That dinner didn't sit well at all—Tom threw up all night after it. The emergency Cipro antibiotic Steffanie had packed didn't help. Neither did gentamicin, which a local doctor infused Tom with the next day. Tom's heart raced, his temperature surged, his blood pressure began to drop, and within hours, he was admitted to a local clinic in critical condition. From there, he was airlifted to Uniklinik, a hospital in Frankfurt, Germany, where the couple's friend Robert "Chip" Schooley, an infectious disease physician at the University of California San Diego, knew some people. And that's where Tom finally got his diagnosis.

A gallstone had blocked his bile duct causing a large abscess to form in his abdomen. But that wasn't all. The abscess was infected with a nightmare superbug called *Acinetobacter baumannii*.

Inside Tom's body, *A. baumannii* formed what doctors call a *pseudocyst*—a sac filled with fluids, enzymes, blood, and the bacteria itself. The doctor who broke the bad news to Steffanie was gravely concerned not only about Tom but about the hospital itself—he worried about the spread of the infection. "I regret to tell you that our microbiology lab has now cultured the sample from the pseudocyst," he told Steffanie, who later recounted the conversation in her book, *The Perfect Predator*. "The pseudocyst is infected with the worst bacteria on the planet. *Acinetobacter baumannii*. This microbe has been responsible for the closure of several ICUs across Europe in recent months. It is the worst news we could have had."[2]

In pictures, *A. baumannii* looks like pink cotton balls that belong in a Barbie dollhouse rather than a biosafety lab. Fuzzy and fluffy, they appear plump and squishy. They may look soft, but they have a very tough skin. Unlike other, more sensitive bacteria, *A. baumannii* flaunts a second coat, a protective capsule stitched together from carbohydrate molecules that shield it from environmental harms. Think of it as a microbial hazmat suit. It helps retain water, keeping the bug nicely hydrated and healthy. It protects the germ from antibiotics. It is also somewhat slippery, so the immune system cells that normally gobble up foreign invaders have trouble grasping it. "The coat is kind of slimy," explains Schooley, the UCSD infectious disease physician. "It makes it hard for the white blood cells to grab it and eat it." Plus, the highly varied *A. baumannii* sports about 150 different types of this goopy, slippery hazmat suit,[3] which makes it even more difficult to deal with.

It gets worse. *A. baumannii* is an expert at picking up antibiotic-resistance genes from other bacterial brethren and filing them into its own genome, like an arsenal of arms. It forms biofilms—microbial commonwealths that allow the bugs to persist through challenging conditions. And even when some specialized antibiotics manage to chip away at the biofilms or at the protective capsule, they don't make much of a dent. *A. baumannii* spits them right out before they do any damage—another clever trick it mastered thanks to the helpful new genes. It can even metabolize some of our wonder drugs as food. A hardy soil bacterium that evolved in the conditions of fierce biological warfare where every microorganism is fighting for survival by poisoning its neighbor with toxins and digesting anything it can grab, *A. baumannii* can gobble certain antibiotics for breakfast.[4] Compared to tough soil conditions, Tom's body was a five-star hotel in which the superbug made a comfortable pseudocyst home and settled in for good.

From her early days at the lab bench, Steffanie remembered working with *A. baumannii* samples. Back then, there was no sense of danger. A common microbe found in soil, water, and plants, *A.*

baumannii had evolved alongside humans and been fairly benign. But that has since changed. Because *A. baumannii* dwells on each and every imaginable surface, including in hospitals and ICUs, it had plenty of time and opportunities to evolve. And so it did. The bug's newer strains picked up antibiotic-resistant genes, outcompeting even the most powerful medicines. One recent report estimated that *A. baumannii* caused 8,500 infections and 700 deaths in just one year in the US alone.[5] Luckily, Tom's acinetobacter isolate showed some sensitivity to three top-gun antibiotics—colistin, meropenem, and tigecycline. That meant that Tom had a chance.

Steffanie and Schooley believed his best chance at survival was on his home turf, at the University of California Thornton Hospital, now called Jacobs Medical Center in San Diego. So in mid-December 2015, Tom was flown to Thornton, where an ICU room became his home for the next several months. Steffanie was optimistic, expecting him to be home for Christmas. But *A. baumannii* snuggling in his pseudocyst had other plans.

Doctors were hesitant to cut the pseudocyst out so instead, they inserted a drain, steadily siphoning out the infection, and then reran the lab tests to see which top-gun antibiotics would still work against the bacteria. The test results were horrifying. *A. baumannii* had evolved to shrug off all three antibiotics—colistin, meropenem, and tigecycline. As a measure of last resort, Tom's doctors began trying different mixes of the trio, hoping to find a synergistic combination that could still fight the superbug.[6]

Before they found any promising combinations, the crisis worsened. Tom's drain slipped, spilling the infectious soup into his insides. Colonized all over his body, he headed straight into sepsis, once again at the brink of death, with no weapons left in the doctors' arsenal. If Steffanie wanted her husband to live, she had to find an alternative herself. She dove into it headfirst, plowing through each and every bit of medical literature she could find.

That was when Steffanie stumbled upon phages. Bacteria had their own enemy, she found, which in the past, had been used to destroy it. She dug up d'Hérelle's original studies. She read about the George Eliava Institute of Bacteriophages, Microbiology and Virology. She found that phages were widely used in the Soviet Union and some Eastern European countries. She even unearthed the information about the FDA's approval of Intralytix's listeria phages for disinfecting meat. And she came across a recent paper by a Georgian scientist, Maya Merabishvili, who assembled a cocktail of phages for burn wounds in Belgium.[7] "I had no idea that phages could be used to treat bacterial infections in people, but the idea was brilliant," she would later write in her book. Now all she needed to do was try to find some phages that preyed on *A. baumannii*. Where did one find therapeutic phages?

In the United States, it seemed, there were no places to contact. There were no approved protocols, no clinical trials, not even cases of compassionate use in which the FDA grants an exception to try an experimental Investigational New Drug, or eIND, because the patient has nothing to lose. But then a colleague told her about a friend who had flown to Tbilisi for a MRSA treatment—and it worked. Steffanie sent Schooley some of the scientific papers she had found. "I know it sounds a little woo woo," she wrote, "but it may be worth a shot."

To Schooley, Steffanie's idea didn't seem outlandish at all. Years earlier, when he first studied medicine, he chose to become an infectious disease scientist because he was interested in antibiotic discovery. But he quickly realized that the antibiotic discoveries were essentially nonexistent, so he switched gears and became a virologist. "We've had very few breakthroughs in new antibiotics for the last thirty years," Schooley says. "So given where we were with Tom's care, it was clear to me that we weren't going to suddenly have a new antibiotic discovery that would change his course. But I know a lot about viruses, and I knew about bacteriophages. I thought it was worth a try." He wasn't worried about giving Tom an experimental phage treatment. He was worried about not finding the right phages fast enough. "I thought it was unlikely that we could find phages in time to save him because he was so ill," Schooley recalls, but he saluted the concept.[8]

"It's an incredibly interesting idea that would be worth thinking about although it might be slightly ahead of its time," he wrote back to Steffanie. To try it out, they first had to find phages that killed this particular superbug. Second, the FDA would have to green-light the phages with an eIND on a onetime basis. "If you can find some phages with activity against the acinetobacter," Schooley wrote, "I will give the FDA a call to see if they will issue an eIND for compassionate use."[9]

Could she find phages that killed the worst bug on the planet? Steffanie embarked on the quest, sending emails to every phage lab and scientist she could find.

The next morning, her inbox was full of replies, none of which were of any use. Most labs didn't stock *A. baumannii* phages. Others politely said that this had never been tried before in humans and wasn't ready to be tested yet. But the very last email offered a glimmer of hope.[10]

THE PHAGE CONVERT

The night Steffanie sent off her emails, Ryland Young was working late in his lab at Texas A&M University. It was around 10:30 p.m. when he wrapped up his experiments and checked his email one last time before heading home. Steffanie's email caught his eye. It mentioned his news comment on phage hunting, which he had said was easy to do, and recounted Tom's harrowing battle with the superbug.[11] "His condition is deteriorating because the infection cannot be controlled and we are considering less conventional approaches," Steffanie wrote. "I recognize that your lab primarily does *in vitro* research, but I am wondering if you have any suggestions for us in terms of phage treatment. Many thanks for considering this unusual request."

Years earlier, Young would likely have replied that the phage therapy wasn't a possibility and sent his regrets. Like most scientists, he had read all the damning 1930s reports and viewed phages as research subjects only. He'd spent over four decades studying phages and never tried using them to save somebody's life. But by 2016, he was a convert. A few years before, he had served on an advisory board of a budding phage therapy start-up, GangaGen, based in India. The start-up had been founded by a retired bio-pharma executive who was inspired by the BBC documentary filmed years earlier at the ill-fated conference at the Eliava Institute in Tbilisi. Young didn't stay in the role long, but that experience changed his view of his research subjects. "The idea of using phages as medicines was always laughed at and ridiculed, and I used to be in that camp," he says, "but that experience changed my thinking. When Steffanie's email came, I was kind of primed for it."[12]

He emailed saying that he was sorry for Tom's situation and offered help finding phages for his acinebacter strains. "Send me Tom's isolates," he told Steffanie on the phone. "We have some phages for *A. baumannii* in our lab, and I will ask other labs to send me theirs," he added. "And we'll also go out looking for more."

After the conversation, Young walked into his lab where two people, a student and a technician, were going about their normal workdays. Young sat them down and explained the situation. A man was dying, and their research could save him. If it worked, of course. "I hadn't even finished my speech, and they were already running to the incubators," he recalls. They had to test so many variations of bacteria and phages that they worked in shifts 24-7, and the equipment was running nonstop. "From that point on, one of them was always in the lab."[13]

Young had some logistical hurdles to overcome too. He needed to inform his Texas A&M leadership of the unconventional project he had embarked on. That was no joke. A dreaded superbug that had defeated every known antibiotic and shut down hospital wards was being sent to a campus of forty thousand students. The superbug was going to be grown in a lab, located in a building that held about two thousand people daily. Young had to convince his biosafety committees and others in charge that the endeavor was safe and sane. One conversation stuck with him. A man recited Young's idea back to him this way: "You want to make a virus cocktail that's unapproved for a therapeutic application, and you're going to do it using Texas A&M facilities, and you're going to send it to a hospital that's going to formulate it and inject it into a person who's probably going to die anyway." "That's the plan," Young answered affirmatively. The university gave him the go-ahead.[14]

In the meantime, Schooley contacted the FDA, which has a specific process for emergency eIND approval, which begins with calling an 800 number. On the other side of the line, an FDA scientist fields these requests—some promising and well researched, and others less so. On the day Schooley dialed the number, the scientist on call was senior regulatory reviewer Cara Fiore, a microbiologist very familiar with the antibiotic resistance threat. "Her brother is an infectious disease specialist who works with the CDC," Schooley shares. "She was well aware of all the difficulties we have when treating people with multidrug resistant infections."[15]

It was hard not to be aware. The resistance threat was surging worldwide, and fast. India was struggling with multidrug-resistant tuberculosis.[16] VRE was rising in Europe.[17] So was *A. baumannii*, which had closed several European hospital wards. In 2011, a superbug version of *Klebsiella pneumoniae* struck really close to home: the NIH Clinical Center had an outbreak of carbapenem-resistant klebsiella that sickened eighteen patients and killed eleven of them.[18] On the CDC's most recent antibiotic resistance report, the stubborn acinetobacter was listed as a "serious threat."[19]

In a rare stroke of luck, Fiore also happened to have a favorable view of bacteriophages. She was familiar with their medicinal potential from the time she worked on her dissertation at the University of Maryland School of Medicine. "The lab where I did my PhD also did phage therapy research," she says. "So my exposure to bacteriophage therapy goes back into the nineties."[20] Fiore listened to Schooley's description of Tom's ordeal, the acinetobacter defeating every medicine they tried, and the plan to sic phages onto it as a last resort. With emergency requests, the agency weighs the severity of the illness, the gravity of the situation, and the chance of saving a human life. "That really sounds interesting; let's see if we can make this work," Schooley recalls Fiore's response. "If you can find phages, we should talk quickly about whether they're in a state to be administered," she added, referring to the fact that phages had to be purified from any toxins that could kill Tom rather than save him.[21]

To Schooley, it sounded like a solid plan. "The FDA understood the gravity of the situation, so they were very much supportive of us moving forward," he says. "When you have a severely ill patient like Tom who could have died any minute, they're willing to listen to anything that sounds reasonable to try to save the patient's life. So the FDA was quite inclined to consider this."

Fiore meant what she said. She immediately connected Schooley to an entity that she knew had the phages specifically against the acinetobacter.[22] Steffanie may have thought she left no stone unturned in the phage universe, but there was one big player she didn't know about.

It was the US military. Serendipitously, for the past five years, both the army and the navy had been collecting phages from all over the world. And that amounted to one impressive library of several thousand bacteria eaters.

THE IRAQIBACTER

The Iraq War was a very different type of combat for the US military. Never before had so many American soldiers fought in desert conditions. And that meant very different types of injuries.

In most prior wars, the majority of injuries came from bullet wounds, which usually have small entry points and relatively small contamination from bacterial organisms. "When the bullet enters you, it will take your clothing with it into the wound, and that's the only contamination you get," explains Young, who spent three years in Vietnam. "And the first thing you do when you treat a bullet wound is you get the clothing out." When cleaned and disinfected promptly and properly, the non-life-threatening wounds usually don't become badly infected.

During the Iraq War, however, the vast majority of injuries were caused by explosions, so these wounds were not only large but often covered in soil and sand. Many soldiers also had burn wounds, with dead tissue that served as food for the incoming organisms. The sand blasts caused by improvised explosive devices seeded broken, bleeding, and burnt tissues with massive amounts of nasty soil bacteria, letting them spread wide and penetrate deep. "The enemy didn't realize that, but it was essentially doing biowarfare because the soldiers would end up with resistant infections," Young says. "Every cut gets coated with bacteria-laden soil, and the soil bacteria is the worst possible bacteria to be involved with." Nicknamed "Iraqibacter" and impervious to many antibiotics, *A. baumannii* was the worst of them all. It cost some American soldiers an arm or a leg. "Some would eventually die or have a very miserable life because of the infection that no one can get rid of," Young says.[23]

The military needed a way to fight the Iraqibacter. And serendipitously, it found just the right people to recruit.

In 2010, when Biswajit Biswas was once again looking for a job, he landed at the Naval Medical Research Command Biological Defense Research Directorate, or NMRC BDRD. Hired by the then BDRD director, Alfred Mateczun, Biswas's role originally had nothing to do with the Iraqibacter. He was charged with researching phages against *Bacillus anthracis*, which causes anthrax, as a means of the biological counterattack. "I was working on anthrax phages, and beyond that, nobody was interested in them," Biswas says. But the war still raged on, and wounded soldiers and mariners were still losing arms and legs to the Iraqibacter. One day, Biswas got a call from the wounds department.[24] Could phages be used to kill that superbug?

Biswas knew such phages existed. Moreover, he had recently isolated some from his usual favorite sewage watering holes, even before he had joined the navy. While working at his previous job at Panacea Pharmaceuticals, he had heard that the Department of Defense was giving out small research grants to isolate phages against the dreaded Iraqibacter. "I applied for the grant, and I got about $200,000 to find some phages for *Acinetobacter baumannii*," he says. "I found them very rapidly, but that was it. Nothing happened afterward."[25] Now the wound department was interested. They asked Biswas what they needed to do to make phage therapy work.

"You need to gather a lot of phages from many different places,"

Biswas said, laying out the plan of attack. "Lots and lots of phages from the environment—from different soil, water, sewage, and different parts of the globe—so we can harvest the most diverse phages possible. The more diversity we have, the greater will be the efficiency."[26]

That phage diversity was particularly important in the Iraqi-bacter case because *A. baumannii* is highly variable, thanks to its 150 different hazmat coat types and other tricks. Even within the same exact strain, one can find bugs with slightly different receptors, onto which different phages latch. Scientists call these variations *isolates*. One patient can be infected with one isolate—or several different ones. Worse, sometimes a bug can mutate within a patient, changing its receptor—and then the existing phage would become useless, even if it was efficient in the past. Phages can rejigger their own receptors too, but that may take time, which patients who fight for their lives don't have. "So you get the bacteria from patient A and other bacteria from patient B, and it's the same *A. baumannii*, but you need two different phages to kill that same bacteria," Biswas explains. "*A. baumannii* is so highly variant that no single phage can cover more than fifty percent of its clinical isolates. You need a diverse group of phages to control them. So I told the wound department that they need to create a phage library." He mentioned that Carl Merril touted that idea before he retired. The navy wanted to talk to Merril too. Biswas looped in his old boss.[27]

"The navy invited me to lunch," Merril recalls. He went for a conversation starter, but shortly after that lunch, the navy lab moved farther away, and he didn't feel like driving that distance. "So I asked them to come over to my house, and we started meeting here, right in my little conference room. And every time, more and more people showed up."[28] Merril explained his phage library vision and why phage cocktails would work. Some navy scientists weren't fully convinced. "I remember one of them said, 'Well, even if we gather a lot of phages, we'll still eventually get resistance to anything we find,'" Merril says. "And I said, 'Yes, but the library would have to be open-ended and we would keep adding more.'" He cited one of his favorite phage statistics. "There are ten to the power of thirty-one of them on the planet. We won't run out of that anytime soon."

The conversations progressed to a formal lecture that the navy asked Merril to give at Walter Reed National Military Medical Center. "They said, 'This time, you should wear a jacket and tie, because there will be a few more people there,'" he recalls. He ended up addressing an auditorium of about two hundred people,[29] with a formal photograph afterward. "They all seemed to be genuinely interested," Merril recalls. "So I outlined exactly how to do this, how to build a phage library. But I had no idea whether they were actually putting everything I said into action."[30]

Meanwhile, the military took Merril's words to heart and launched a massive campaign to gather phages from all over the world. Wherever the navy ships went and wherever the army was stationed, recruits, lieutenants, and even colonels dipped buckets in dirty waters, muddy streams, gunky sewage, and cow feces. "Anyplace your ships go, grab some samples," Biswas told commanders. "Any phages are good phages." Soon samples began to arrive from Peru, Ghana, Thailand, Egypt, and Cambodia. A few were picked from the local hospitals because that's where antibiotic-resistant bugs commonly dwell, along with the phages that devour them. Over a few years, the military amassed several thousand bacteria eaters—a collection that likely would have made the 1960s Soviet Ministry of Health jealous. All phages were meticulously cataloged and filed away in freezers, floating in tiny vials, and waiting for an opportune moment to unleash their lytic wrath.

That moment came when Cara Fiore told Chip Schooley about them.

THE SUPERBUG STANDOFF

Schooley got off the phone frustrated and disheartened. He just spent a long time talking to the army and the navy, both of which confirmed that they had the phages against the Iraqibacter, but they weren't in a hurry to send them. "We aren't in the business of civilian medicine," said the army representative. Safety, he said, was their primary concern—they didn't want to use an untested substance on a dying person and become a media scapegoat afterward. The phages weren't going to be available. Schooley couldn't understand that attitude. He had spoken to the Belgian officers who offered to send their phages in a diplomatic pouch. "If the Belgian military could do it, why couldn't ours?" he asked.

Schooley didn't know it, but he was not the only person unhappy with the conversation. Theron Hamilton, the navy representative who kept quiet during the call, was equally dissatisfied. "We're a military organization, and we have a mandate and a mission to serve our military personnel, which makes perfect sense," he says. "But when you're in the business of doing applied research, which you are funding with taxpayer dollars, I believe that you have an obligation to the taxpayer and to the citizens of the United States to do all you can, if you have a resource available." Hamilton thought it over and called Schooley back. He explained that he would have to get permission from several superior officers, but he was willing to give it a try. "Send the isolates," he told Schooley, "and we'll see what we can do."[31]

Hamilton also had strong reasons to believe that phages would work. He was very familiar with the concept because he was the head of the lab where Biswajit Biswas worked. He had seen the phages' "tailwork" in action, so to him, denying someone such a strong lifesaving chance was simply wrong. "So my goal was to ensure that we use this resource on an American citizen and make sure that we got all of the proper permissions to do so."

Tom's isolates arrived the next day, and Hamilton went around to secure the proper permission, which ultimately came from the center's director, Alfred Mateczun, who had originally hired Biswas. Mateczun listened to Hamilton's description of Schooley's request and made sure he understood the situation. "We have the bacteria and the phage that will kill it?" he asked. Hamilton replied affirmatively. "Send the phage," Mateczun said. For the next couple of weeks, Hamilton's lab worked night and day, combing their collection for the right phages.

With that, the fight to save Tom with phage therapy became the first truly global effort transcending all borders and boundaries, as science should. The US military was testing out phages from the remotest corners of the world. Young's team was digging through the dirtiest places imaginable—sewage streams as well as cowsheds and pigsties in College Station, Texas. The Belgian military sent their bacteria eaters. Maya Merabishvili, originally from Georgia but working in Belgium, whose study Steffanie found online, advised on phage dosing. So did Carl Merril.

Once the teams found the phages that destroyed *A. baumannii* and began growing them, there came the next step: removing the leftover toxins so that Tom wouldn't go into shock. With *A. baumannii*, it was a particularly intricate challenge. The bug's slimy outer coat is covered with lipopolysaccharide molecules, which become the so-called endotoxin when the bacteria fall apart—and that causes the immune system to go into a potentially lethal overdrive.[32]

Young's team had a moment of panic when they measured the endotoxin level in their already-purified brew—it was still sky-high. "We were horrified by the high level of endotoxin even after the purification," he says. "We never had to clean phages for our lab experiments, so we had no way of purifying them further." Luckily, a specialized lab at San Diego State University was able to do it with a top-notch centrifuge. On the navy side, it was Carl Merril who purified the phages with the same techniques he learned during his university days at Cold Spring Harbor Laboratory—also using a centrifuge. The Texas four-phage cocktail arrived first—Young's team beat the navy's crew by a couple of days because they had an earlier start.

That first phage mix was to be infused into Tom's abdomen rather than into his bloodstream. The doctors agreed that this was a safer bet. An intravenous administration could draw a much more violent response from his immune system. If Tom lived through the infusion experiment, he would probably live through the intravenous one.

The procedure, performed on March 15, drew a crowd of medics, all of whom gathered around Tom's bed. Fiore, who was based in Maryland, called Schooley from her son's hockey game to check in. The hospital's pharmacist, who received the phages, brought them into Tom's room in a foam box where they were kept at 4°C (39.2°F). The attending physician filled the syringes with the phage brew and emptied them into the drains that so far had been syphoning A. baumannii out of Tom.[33] The "Texas tea," as Steffanie called it, had been administered. Tom received a dose every two hours. Over the next forty-eight hours, he suffered no adverse reactions.

Two days later, Tom received the intravenous four-phage navy cocktail. His emaciated body didn't react to the living medicines pouring into his veins whatsoever. "It was anticlimactic," Steffanie would write later. And yet, it was the riskiest moment because no one knew how Tom would react. And for the first twenty-four hours, he didn't react at all.

A day later, he woke up, after more than three months in a coma.

He was conscious for a brief moment, enough to recognize his daughter, lift his head off the pillow, give a nod—and fall back to sleep. On March 22, he was awake enough that he tried to pull the ventilator tube out of his throat and mouthed, "Water." A few days later, when he was strong enough to breathe on his own, doctors took him off the ventilator.

But the superbug wasn't done with him yet. By April 1, his fever spiked and his blood pressure began to drop. The *A. baumannii* didn't want to leave, so it pulled yet another genetic trick.

Ever since the phage cocktails arrived, the *A. baumannii* was losing ground. The phages, formulated specifically to attack the isolates ravaging Tom's insides, excelled at clinging to the specific receptors on the bacteria's surface and slipping inside it. Even the bugs' elaborately varied goopy coat didn't help. In fact, that coat had become a problem, a liability to the bacteria's survival. And so the microorganism did the most logical thing possible: it dropped its coat.

Described in scientific terms, *A. baumannii* mutated again and shed its once-protective capsule. It switched into an un-capsulated form.

With that capsule, out went all the receptors the phages used to latch on to the bug. For a while, the phages kept killing the remaining, unmutated acinetobacter brethren. But the new mutants, unchecked and impervious to the phages, began to multiply rapidly—and they once again overpowered Tom's immune system. When Hamilton received Tom's new isolates, the new *A. baumannii* population was resistant to all phages in both cocktails, except one. But that one fighter couldn't keep up with the rising mutant *A. baumannii* population. Tom needed new phages that could prey on the un-capsulated mutants. To Biswas, that genetic game made perfect sense. "If you're only using the phage that works on the capsulated version, you will kill all the capsulated bacteria, but the un-capsulated ones will have an open field and multiply uncon-trollably," he says.[34]

And so Biswas's group packed up and ventured out to their favorite sewage watering holes. Once again, they dipped the buck-ets into the swirling brown stream. Once again, they brought the spoils of their trip back to the lab. Once again, they isolated phages from the goo and pitted them against the *A. baumannii*. And they found the new phage.

The slayer of mutant *A. baumannii* was different. It was shorter and stockier than its cousins, which destroyed the previous ver-sions of the acinetobacter in Tom's body. In the bacteria eaters' no-menclature of that time, such short phages were called *podophages*, while their longer relatives were named *myophages*.[35] The squatty newfound podophage had a very short tail, but it worked won-ders with it. Not only did it effectively attack the un-capsulated mutants, but it destroyed Tom's original *A. baumannii* equally well. And it was a good team player too. It worked synergistically with one of its cousins from Tom's original cocktail and with an antibiotic called minocycline. Dubbed the Super Killer, the short podophage helped extinguish the superbug from Tom's body.[36]

From that point on, Tom took a steady path to recovery. He was home a few months later. The couple's ordeal with the worst bacteria on the planet was winding down, but the mark they have made in the field of phage therapy was just beginning. Stirred by the perfect storm of Tom and Steffanie's experience, the living medicines' paradigm was going to change greatly in the next few years.

14

The Perfect Storm's Aftermath

In February 2018, when winter was still in full swing, a long-anticipated paper finally landed on Sandro's desk. It was an approval for a clinical trial that involved bacteriophage preparation. Intralytix would be growing bacteriophages to tackle Crohn's disease—a chronic inflammation of the gastrointestinal tract that causes pain, diarrhea, fatigue, weight loss, and malnutrition, and has no known cure.

When the approval arrived, Sandro popped a bottle of champagne and toasted with his entire crew of about twenty people. Things had finally turned around for his start-up. And for his phages too. It took two decades, but Sandro felt that he had at last transcended what appeared to be an impassable wall.

The first clinical trial breakthrough for Intralytix was in the making for some time. A few years earlier, Sandro got a call from Ferring Pharmaceuticals, a Swiss pharmaceutical company. Started by Frederik and Eva Paulsen in 1950 and at the time led by Frederik Paulsen Jr., the company retained a family-owned spirit and a keen interest in niche therapies. Ferring's portfolio focused mostly on maternal and infant wellness. "Ferring had nothing to do with infectious diseases or with phages per se," Sandro says. "They're very active in reproductive health, women's health, gut health, and those types of things. So normally, they wouldn't be on a list of contacts that I would be reaching out to, and it was a little unexpected to get a call from them. But they wanted to talk to me."[1]

Things became clear after the first conversation. Ferring was interested in trying phages to treat Crohn's. Crohn's existing treatments aim to minimize symptoms and keep the disease in remission as much as possible, but there is no cure. Antibiotics help some people, but the symptoms usually come back after time. Some very recalcitrant cases are treated with chemotherapy, which often has harmful side effects. Others are treated with surgery, in which the inflamed portion of the intestines are cut out, but the disease almost always returns, striking a different part of the gut. Repeated surgeries diminish patients' ability to absorb nutrients from food. Some Crohn's sufferers end up having to wear a colostomy bag because they lose so much of their intestines to the inflammation.[2]

About one in every one hundred Americans battle Inflammatory Bowel Disease, which includes Crohn's,[3] but its origins are still a mystery. One theory is that Crohn's is an autoimmune condition, in which the body's own immune system attacks the stomach lining, mistakenly triggered by bacteria in the digestive tract. A different view holds that the immune system does in fact have an enemy to battle, but it is unable to extinguish it, so the inflammation becomes chronic. Recent studies linked Crohn's to the presence of the adherent invasive *E. coli*, which seems to persist in the guts of Crohn's sufferers, but not in healthy people.[4]

Paulsen wanted to find phages to work against the invasive *E. coli* and target specifically that bacteria while leaving all other legitimate gut dwellers intact. He understood how phages worked. So he tasked his staff with finding suitable phage collaborators.

Ferring's first move was to speak to the Pasteur Institute in Paris. From there, the company had obtained some phages that indeed worked against the adherent invasive *E. coli*. Now Ferring needed a company that could manufacture them. The Pasteur Institute isn't in the business of drug development, so Ferring started looking for companies in the phage world.

Serendipitously, Paulsen was familiar with Eliava Institute and its tumultuous history. Even better, he was fond of Georgia. "He owns a few properties there," says Sandro—including the iconic Château Mukhrani, a nineteenth-century palace in Georgia's wine country. "His son lives in Georgia. He was intrigued by Georgians and by phages too." But rather than heading east, he wanted to bring his product to the American market. Intralytix had the best of both worlds—located in America yet connected to Georgia's decades of phage wisdom—and so Sandro got the call.

Ferring wanted Intralytix to grow phages for the adherent invasive *E. coli* and work with the FDA to green-light a clinical trial. The Swiss company had the money to back the effort while Intralytix had the years of experience of working with the FDA on phages for food sprays. The two soon embarked on the joint venture.

The progress was slow. Ferring wanted to adhere to the strictest production methods per the Good Manufacturing Practice (GMP) standards. Intralytix's facilities weren't set up for the medical-grade production. Ferring wanted Sandro to find a company with GMP facilities and work with it to grow phages.

The problem was that, at the time, no pharmaceutical company knew how to manufacture phages, and most *didn't want* to make them. Some were downright afraid to deal with them. Many pharma and biotech companies use nonpathogenic *E. coli* to generate therapeutic proteins for various disorders, which are harvested and turned into medicines. They didn't want to introduce *E. coli* slayers into their facilities. "They were afraid the phages would kill their workhorse organism and stop their main production," Sandro says. It was a risky proposition. "No one wanted to take the chance."[5]

After months of searching, he found one company, but the price was astronomical. "They quoted us a six-million-dollar price to make one liter of phage," he says—a quarter of a gallon. "So obviously, we laughed and continued looking. After several months, we found another one that gave us a price of one-point-five million for the same amount. It was still mind-boggling."

For his part, Sandro didn't think that the strict medical-grade rules were needed just yet. Clinical trials usually go through three phases. "The FDA doesn't require GMP standards for phase 1 clinical trials," he says. It makes it so expensive that most ideas would never be tested.

After the fruitless two-year-long quest, Sandro finally convinced Ferring to let Intralytix do the job. "It's a big company with a lot of different committees, so it took time," he says. "But the FDA confirmed that GMP wasn't required for the phase 1 trial. So I told Ferring, 'Let us do it. We are small, we are nimble, we can get it done fast.'" He got the long-awaited go-ahead from the committees, found a clinical partner at Mount Sinai Hospital in New York, put the paperwork together, and sent it off to the FDA.[6]

In early 2018—two decades after he formed his company with the goal of making living medicines—the first clinical trial approval had arrived.

With that encouragement, Sandro put together the next proposal—to test phages against shigella—and sent it off to NIH, asking for funding. After that, he revived the idea that started it all—using phages to treat VRE. Over the next couple of years, the FDA gave him a thumbs-up for both. "We spent twenty years educating the FDA about phages, and it finally paid off," Sandro says. "We consistently demonstrated that our phages were safe, that they worked, and that the bacteria didn't develop resistance. All that laid the groundwork for medical applications, which was our original goal. It took a long time, but we made it there."

The world's infectious disease situation had changed too. In the 1990s, when Glenn Morris and Sandro first approached the regulatory agencies to test phage treatments for VRE, the antibiotic-resistant menace was relatively low and optimism about new antibiotics was reasonably high. By the second decade of the new millennium, the threat was not just pressing but hanging over the medical community like an axe about to fall.

The CDC's report on antibiotic resistance published in 2013 was damning. It estimated that two million Americans each year fall ill with antibiotic-resistant infections, and at least twenty-three thousand die as a result. It also added that in reality, these numbers were likely higher because some cases are not reported. With twelve germs listed as serious threats, the multidrug-resistant *Acinetobacter* took the front seat, followed by other familiar culprits like MRSA and VRE, and joined by some newer variants like drug-resistant shigella and salmonella.[7]

Scientists sounded the alarm that humankind was entering a post-antibiotic era, and they weren't far from the truth. In April 2015, only months before Tom Patterson fell ill, another report came out revealing that the antibiotic pipelines were running dry. "Of the 18 largest pharmaceutical companies, 15 abandoned the antibiotic field," the report stated, listing multiple reasons for this alarming development. One was the lack of economic incentive—antibiotic discovery and development took years, millions of dollars, lengthy clinical trials, and little return on investment. Compared to maintenance drugs for blood pressure or diabetes that patients take daily, most people use antibiotics for a very short time—days or weeks—so the companies do not sell enough, especially considering the unpredictable but inevitable outcome of antibiotic resistance. The financial collapse of 2008 exacerbated the trend. When some pharmaceutical companies merged in the meltdown's aftermath, they scaled down on the less lucrative medications. At the same time, research in academia shrank due to lack of funding.[8]

The two reports made one thing obvious: humans desperately needed new antimicrobial weapons. So regulatory agencies began investigating alternatives. Phages came back on the scene shortly after the 2011 carbapenem-resistant klebsiella outbreak killed eleven patients in the NIH Clinical Center, says Joseph Campbell, program officer at the Research Resources section at NIAID. "After the outbreak, some scientists began asking NIAID to support development of phages so that if it happened again, phages could be an option," he says. "That started a bacteriophage interest group, and then we started meeting with the FDA."[9] And then there came the perfect storm: Patterson's case that finally brought change.

That change did not happen when Sandro and Glenn first put together their VRE proposal in the mid-1990s. It didn't happen when Caisey Harlingten brought a crowd of phage researchers together in Tbilisi shortly thereafter. It didn't happen when Carl Merril floated the idea of a phage library. But it finally did happen in 2016, reviving phages' reputation as potent antibiotic alternatives. By then, the time was right.

"The FDA reviews all of the antibiotic applications, and they're just as aware as all the rest of us that there isn't much coming out of the antibiotic pipeline. In fact, they're more aware of it than we are because they see all the applications before we do," Schooley says. By 2016, the agency *had been waiting* for a Patterson-like situation to happen, he shares. "They had been looking for a case that was urgent enough to move forward with and had been worked up well enough that we could at least treat the patient and have some idea about what would happen." The FDA *wanted* to see this approach tried, Schooley points out. "Regardless of the outcome," he adds.[10]

And the outcome beat all expectations. With Patterson's recovery, phages finally and firmly earned their place among other respectable biological medicines. The FDA now regulates phages under its Center for Biologics Evaluation and Research (CBER) group, of which Fiore is a part. "The FDA uses its scientific and regulatory expertise to facilitate phage development," she says.[11]

Within the last few years, the phage therapy research field has blossomed. The NIAID funded several phage therapy research projects. The FDA green-lighted a number of compassionate use cases. Phage researchers who studied basic phage biology began to apply their knowledge to devise lifesaving therapeutics. Phage labs opened, aiming to translate research into medicinal applications. In 2017, the agency hosted a workshop on bacteriophage therapy for researchers interested in pursuing it. It followed up with another one in 2021. "The purpose of these workshops is to discuss the scientific and regulatory considerations for bacteriophage therapy and provide a forum for the exchange of information and perspectives," Fiore says. "We closely collaborate with NIH, academia, and industry."[12]

Together with other colleagues, Steffanie Strathdee and Schooley formed the Center for Innovative Phage Applications and Therapeutics, or IPATH, at the University of California San Diego in 2018. IPATH describes its goal as pursuing "through collaboration with researchers, companies and institutions around the world, new treatments for combating antimicrobial resistant diseases."

IPATH has run only six clinical trials so far,[13] but in addition to its main goals to treat patients and test phage in clinical trials, it also disseminates information on how to get access to therapy and move the field forward, says Strathdee. "Because of the publicity around my husband's case, people are coming to me personally," she says. "So I get involved in helping patients to determine whether they are going to be eligible for phage therapy. I would enlist the help of Chip and others and, if they thought that the FDA would probably grant an eIND, we would reach out to labs."

At the same time, a number of phage start-ups have burgeoned in Europe, North America, and beyond, each with their own research and commercializing strategy. To stay in business, pharmaceutical companies rely on patents for the inventions. But because it is not possible to patent natural organisms, phages aren't patentable. To be competitive, companies must figure out how to stake the claim on their inventions and be profitable.

Some, like Sandro, are patenting cocktails of natural phages, which are highly effective against specific infections. Others are genetically modifying their phages to make them more efficient. "We believe in payloads, in engineering the virus to carry something that helps improve its natural killing efficacy," says Paul Garofolo, CEO and cofounder of Locus Biosciences, which uses CRISPR technology to give their living medicines an extra punch. Genetically engineered phages are patentable, which is one reason why Locus Biosciences attracted top pharmaceutical investors and funding. "In our minds, that is what a phage needs in order to effectively compete with the replacement of antibiotics," Garofolo says. Yet others see phages and antibiotics complementing each other and being administered together.[14]

Similarly to Intralytix, other players in the phage universe have also started clinical trials. Locus Biosciences, for example, started one for urinary tract infections. Adaptive Phage Therapeutics has launched trials for tissue and bone infections. Paul Turner, professor of ecology and evolutionary biology at Yale University, has already finished a small phase 1 trial for cystic fibrosis, a lung disease that makes people susceptible to bacterial infections. Today, ClinicalTrials.gov lists a flurry of trials in different stages. Each with their own focus, angle, and modus operandi, these efforts are tackling a spectrum of stubborn infections. "I'm just glad the paradigm has finally shifted," Sandro says. "Because we will save a lot more lives that way. And we'll improve the quality of life for many, many people."

In the few years since Patterson's perfect storm, various phage therapy efforts proved that they could work when all else failed. And the global phage movement finally began to take off, reaching far and wide.

SAVING THE LUNG TRANSPLANT TEEN

One day in spring 2018, Graham Hatfull, professor of biotechnology at the University of Pittsburgh, received a call from a colleague in London, James Soothill from the Great Ormond Street Hospital. "Would you happen to have some phages against the mycobacterium in your collection?" Soothill asked.

Hatfull had spent decades studying phages, but he did basic science research. His work didn't revolve around any clinical applications. As a postdoc at Cambridge, Hatfull worked with twice Nobel laureate Frederick Sanger, a biochemist who developed gene-sequencing techniques. When he came to the University of Pittsburgh in 1988, Hatfull began sequencing phages and comparing their genomes to study their origins and evolutions. The first bacteriophage he sequenced was the one for the infectious mycobacterium. He went on to sequence more and, as the technology grew cheaper, launched a unique program that allowed college and high school students to do real-life biology work. Students, some local and others in faraway locations, would hunt for phages in the woods, bogs, muddy streams, and other places. They isolated the phages, named them, sequenced their genomes, and uploaded the information to a shared database. By the time Hatfull got the call, the program, called SEA-PHAGES (Science Education

Alliance–Phage Hunters Advancing Genomics and Evolutionary Science) had accumulated about fifteen thousand different bacteria eaters, all neatly labeled and stored in the University of Pittsburgh's freezers, as well as at other schools too. Today, Hatfull's collection numbers about twenty-two thousand specimens.

"Not all of them are sequenced, but about forty-five hundred of them are," Hatfull says, "which provides a really superb dataset for understanding how phage genomes differ from each other, what kinds of genes they carry, how they've evolved and all of those basic science types of questions." He most certainly had plenty of phages for the mycobacterium, but what was it for?

Soothill filled him in. A teenage girl in London was fighting a mycobacterium infection in her lungs, and she didn't have long to live.

Isabelle Holdaway was born with cystic fibrosis, a progressive genetic disease that causes the lungs to fill with thick mucus that blocks airways, leads to lung damage, and increases susceptibility to germs. Patients with cystic fibrosis are very prone to lung infections, and Isabelle had been battling one since she was eight years old. By the time she was fourteen, her lungs operated at less than a third of normal capacity. Her doctors decided that a lung transplant would be the best option.

Her operation went well, but afterward, an antibiotic-resistant *Mycobacterium abscessus*, a distant cousin of the tuberculosis-causing blight, took hold. Transplant patients' bodies commonly reject the new organs because their immune systems see them as foreign. To avoid that, patients must take immunosuppressants, which undermine the body's natural infection-fighting abilities. Under those conditions, *M. abscessus* spread through Isabelle's entire body, infecting her liver and her surgical wound and forming lesions on her skin. A few months after the transplant, Isabelle was completely colonized by the germ. She was sent home from the hospital on palliative care. Her mother read about phage therapy online and pleaded with doctors to give it a try. Soothill thought of Hatfull.

The two men had met years earlier at the phage conference in Tbilisi organized by Caisey Harlingten. The guests were drinking champagne with BBC cameramen buzzing around, and the two researchers discussed what could evolve from that effervescent event. Now, years later, Soothill remembered that Hatfull had sequenced the mycobacterium phage and had a few thousand others in his collection. "There's evidence that phage therapy works, and we'd like to try it," Soothill said on the phone.

Hatfull considered himself a basic science microbiologist. "For most of my career, I haven't done much that is directly clinical," he says. But after living medicines saved Tom Patterson a year before, their therapeutic potential was promising once again. Hatfull told Soothill to send the strains, even though he had his doubts. "In *Mycobacterium abscessus*, there's enormous variation from strain to strain and patient to patient," he says. "So I was skeptical as to whether we would find phages for these particular strains. And I would say that when we received the strains, I envisaged therapy as being an unlikely outcome."[15]

The strains arrived, and Hatfull's lab began combing through the collection. Soon three promising candidates emerged. Named by the students who discovered them as Muddy, ZoeJ, and BPs, they came not only from different locations but from different continents. Isolated from a rotten eggplant by a student in South Africa during a workshop, Muddy proved to be the best mycobacteria killer. BPs was found in Pittsburgh and ZoeJ at Providence College in Rhode Island, but they performed poorly compared to the mighty Muddy. Multi-phage cocktails are always best to circumvent bacteria's resistance, so Hatfull decided to fine-tune the weaker duo. BPs was trained to attack mycobacteria more effectively by breeding a more potent version—a method not unlike what d'Hérelle outlined in his book. ZoeJ was genetically tweaked—a gene was cut out of its DNA to turn it into an efficient mycobacteria eater.[16] The three phages were grown, purified, and mixed into a cocktail that in June 2018 arrived at Great Ormond Street Hospital in London.

Isabelle was treated with phages every twelve hours for more than seven months. During the first two days, she felt sweaty and flushed, but had no fever. Nine days later, she went home, but continued coming to the hospital for treatments. Over six months, she gradually got healthier. Her liver went back to normal. Her surgical cut and her skin healed, and her lungs were working better. She had no adverse reactions to phages.[17]

Isabelle died a few years later due to an unrelated health issue, but she was the first person in the world to be treated with a phage genetically engineered to improve its performance. Her case inspired others to seek similar treatments. "We've gone quite a long way in terms of doing these compassionate use interventions," Hatfull says. "We have now provided phages for probably thirty-five patients like her, and we've written up a series of case studies of twenty of them."[18]

ON HIS LAST LEG

John Haverty wanted just one more summer. Just one more season to drive his slick BMW Roadster. To mow his lawn. To work in his yard. To just walk around. Then, by Christmas, he would let his leg go. He would submit to the amputation and accept his life as a disabled person. "The only cure is to amputate your leg at the hip," said his doctor. "So when you're ready, come back and we'll do the procedure." Haverty was devastated. "If I could wear a prosthesis afterwards, I'd be okay with it," he says, "but there was no chance of having a prosthetic leg, because it was too high. There'd be nowhere to attach it to." He'd spend the rest of his life in a wheelchair, and he wasn't even sixty yet.

John's medical odyssey began in 2008, when osteoarthritis ate away at his knees, and he needed joint replacements. He was in his late forties, still strong, healthy, and doing things he enjoyed. He was a chef at one of the Mayo Clinic's hospitals in the Midwest. He volunteered as an emergency medical responder. He loved riding a motorcycle and driving his manual BMW Roadster.

Fixing a worn-out knee is one of the most common forms of joint replacement surgeries. They are so routine that over six hundred thousand are done annually in the US.[19] After some recovery time, most people resume their lives, enjoying being able to walk, climb stairs, and play sports again. John had his left knee fixed in March and his right one in November. He thought he had moved on. But then, in early December, barely two weeks after the last surgery, he had an accident.

He was getting out of his Roadster at a gas station when he stepped on a patch of ice. He was still only halfway out of the car, so his left leg went underneath it, and his right got caught in between the steering wheel and the seat. As he fell, the recently operated leg pulled and twisted, so the still-healing incision popped open. "I felt blood streaming down my leg, and I knew I was in trouble," he says. A seasoned EMT, he stopped the bleeding, drove home, and washed up the wound. Then he drove himself to the Mayo Clinic and called his wife, Barbara—a surgical nurse who worked there—to tell her he was coming.

The doctors cleaned the incision and stitched it up again, and John put the episode behind him. But the damage was done. The bacterial menagerie that normally dwells on the skin without causing any trouble had wiggled its way in—and settled for good. Two months later, he was on antibiotics, first pills and then intravenous infusions. When those didn't help, surgeons had to remove his new knee joint, put in a dummy device called a *spacer*, and infuse it with antibiotics to kill the germs. Without the joint, John's leg didn't bend, so he couldn't walk for several weeks, moving around with a walker until doctors deemed the infection cleared and put his artificial knee back. "For a year or two after that, he was fine," Barbara recalls. And then he wasn't again. And again. And again.[20]

Over the years, John went through a total of eighteen surgeries, each of which took a toll on his mental and physical health. He lived on antibiotics, but some didn't work, and others caused severe allergies so he couldn't take them. Several times, he almost went into sepsis. "One time, he thought he had the flu because he wasn't feeling well and had a fever," Barbara says. "And I just happened to see his leg as he got off the couch, and it was so red and swollen that I said, 'Oh my gosh, we have to go to the hospital,' because he was becoming septic." Another time, John woke up in the middle of the night in unbearable pain. His leg had been sore all evening, but now the pain had become excruciating. Walking down the stairs took an hour, and he cried while putting on a shoe. "I am not an emotional guy, but I was in so much pain that I was crying and screaming," he recalls. "I didn't know such pain could exist." Sometime around 2015, he could no longer work in a kitchen and went on disability. By 2018, his surgical cleanups became almost routine. After operating on John four times in a span of two months, his surgeon said this couldn't continue. "At some point, this infection would spread and kill me," John says.

The day after this conversation, as John was still recovering from his latest surgery in the hospital, two infectious disease specialists came to check on him. "Is there anything else we can do?" John asked. "And if I am to lose my leg, can we try some experimental treatment to advance science?" The two medics looked at each other, and one of them uttered the word *bacteriophage*. John listened to their explanations. A university in California was running a small bacteriophage trial John could try applying for. "I'd like to do it," he said.

The doctors submitted John's application, but he was turned down: the study was designed to test one bacteriophage against one bacteria, but John had two proliferating in his leg—klebsiella and enterococcus. So John and Barbara took matters into their own hands. They researched other bacteriophage trials. They called other institutions. They wrote to the Eliava Institute. "We looked at the clinic in the Republic of Georgia, but they don't have the ability to purify it like we do here in the United States," says Barbara. John would need an intravenous, toxin-free bacteriophage, and the Eliava Institute couldn't provide that. Finally, in early 2019, a Maryland-based start-up named Adaptive Phage Therapeutics replied with a lukewarm answer. "We are very busy preparing for clinical trials, but if your doctors send us your isolate, we'll try to find a phage." Barbara thought it was a polite rejection, but John saw it as a foot in the door.

Although barely two years old, Adaptive Phage Therapeutics wasn't exactly a new player in the phage-sphere. It was formed by Carl Merril and his son, Greg. Tom Patterson's case cut Merril's leisurely retirement short. After Tom's spectacular recovery, the military decided to put their extensive phage collection to use. They reached out to pharmaceutical companies, offering their vast library of living medicines. To their surprise, there were no takers. The companies cited the same familiar set of obstacles. Too hard to grow. Too difficult to purify. Too cumbersome to get FDA approval. Too expensive to produce commercially. Too uncertain to take an investment risk. After several unsatisfying attempts, the military approached Carl, who looped in Greg because he had successful experience running a business. "The military licensed their collection to Adaptive Phage Therapeutics," says Greg Merril, the CEO.

In early 2019, a new infectious disease doctor, Gina Suh, joined the Mayo Clinic. With a specialty in musculoskeletal infections, Suh had worked with wounds patients at Stanford Medical Center in Palo Alto and studied phages at Stanford's Bollyky Lab. "I worked in a basic science lab that dealt with phages and it was my dream, or my goal, to bring phages to Mayo," she says. "I had no idea if it was going to be possible or impossible, but I wanted to try it." Then John's case landed on her desk.

John's biggest threat at the time was klebsiella, so Suh sent the isolate to Adaptive Phage Therapeutics. She also filed an eIND with the FDA, which, like Patterson's case, was routed to Cara Fiore.[21] The eIND was approved, and by late spring, the phages arrived. On Friday, June 14, John was scheduled for his first infusion. He was anxious, but optimistic. "My leg was red and swollen again, with fistulas all over and ready to pop. It needed surgery really bad," he recalls. John believed he had nothing to lose. But Barbara, who went with him, was nervous. "We didn't know what the bacteriophage typically does to people," she says. "We didn't know how John was going to react. He had so many bad reactions to antibiotics."

The first infusion took about twenty minutes, and John went home. He received his second the next Monday. That evening, as they sat together at home, Barbara looked at her husband's leg— and did a double take. "Maybe it's my imagination, but I think it looks better," she said cautiously.

"I think it looks better too," John replied. "And it doesn't hurt as bad."

Neither one said much more, unwilling to jinx it. The next morning, as Suh examined John's leg, she had the same reaction. "Doesn't it look better?" Barbara asked.

"I think it does," Suh answered.[22]

If they had doubts, photos taken before and after the start of the infusions confirmed their observations. John's infection was starting to subside. After forty infusions, klebsiella was no longer detectable.

For a while, Suh expected the infection to come back. "I was afraid that it was too good to be true," she says. "Every time I got an email or phone call, I thought, *Oh, the infection is back.* I kept waiting for it to return. And when it became clear that it wasn't, I was completely thrilled. Being able to help somebody like this is a feeling that you keep chasing as a doctor. I want to be able to keep doing that. It has been a major motivation for me to continue working with phages."[23]

A couple of years later, John attempted to use another phage to banish the enterococcus from his troubled leg. But this time, it didn't work as well. Barbara attributes it to the fact that too much time had passed between collecting John's bacterial isolate and growing the phage for it—during the pandemic, everything was slow—and the germ may have mutated by the time the phage brew was ready. Luckily, so far, antibiotics keep John's enterococcus in check, and he is happy with the status quo. "I kept my leg," he says. "I couldn't ask for more."

DODGING THE LUNG TRANSPLANT

Andrey Zvyagintsev lay in a coma so deep his doctors didn't think he would ever come out of it. An antibiotic-resistant strain of klebsiella had colonized his lungs, spread to his other organs, and proliferated in his blood. He was in sepsis and on life support, and no antibiotics at the Institute of Transfusion Medicine and Transplant Engineering in Hannover, Germany, were helping.

A legend of Russian cinematography, Zvyagintsev had won three Cannes Film Festival awards, as well as a long list of others. Born and raised in Novosibirsk, a snowbound Siberian city, he started his acting career in Moscow in the 1990s. For the next three decades, he had a spectacular ascent, equally famous in his home country and in Europe for the emotionally charged, heartbreaking human drama he vividly portrayed in his works. In 2000, he directed his first movie, and three years later, he won the Venice Film Festival's highest prize, the Golden Lion, for the coming-of-age drama *The Return*. In 2007, he received his first Cannes awards for the mind-twisting family tragedy *The Banishment* and four years later his second Cannes award for *Elena*, a crime film he wrote and directed. In 2015, he received a Golden Globe Award for *Leviathan* and three years later the Best Foreign Film by the César Academy for *Loveless*. In that same year, he also served on the Cannes Film Festival jury. Now, his battle with klebsiella was starting to look like his last act.

Zvyagintsev's ordeal with the microscopic rodlike invaders began almost immediately after he battled his way through Covid. When lockdown started in Moscow, he followed the rules, haunted by an uncanny premonition that he was one of the people extremely susceptible to the virus. "It was a gut feeling," he recalls. "I can't explain it, but I just knew it." As soon as the Russian vaccines became available in 2021, he got his shot. Feeling a little better protected, he lowered his guard—it was summer, after all, the perfect time to be outside and outdoors—and contracted Covid almost immediately. He spent the entire month of July in a Moscow hospital, two weeks of it in an ICU, where he beat the blight and came home. Within days, he was back in ICU, his lungs once again infected and inflamed. "We think he picked it up in the hospital," says his wife, Anya. "And because he was so ravaged by Covid, his immune system was also very weak." Worse, he developed a pulmonary embolism—a blood clot that clogged an artery supplying the oxygen flow to his already struggling lungs. Growing worse by the minute, he was spiraling down so fast that his doctor told Anya, "I don't think we will be able to do anything." He suggested they transfer to a European clinic, where Zvyagintsev could get a lung transplant.

On August 15, Zvyagintsev was airlifted to Germany, where doctors first considered clearing his artery, but because the clot was small, they decided against it, recalls Hannover cardiac surgeon Daniel Moskalenko, a Moldovan expat to Germany who grew up watching Zvyagintsev's films and was a passionate fan. "When he arrived, we spent the entire first night talking about movies," says Moskalenko, who helped Anya translate medical lingo during the couple's hospital ordeal. After the first night, he could no longer talk to his favorite film director. Zvyagintsev was running so low on oxygen that he had to be put on a ventilator and in a medically induced coma.[24]

Shortly thereafter, it became clear that even European medicine didn't have any effective weapons against Zvyagintsev's klebsiella strain. The German doctors pumped medicines into him, quickly running through their antibiotics arsenal. When they'd gone through a list of over twenty wonder drugs to no avail, Zvyagintsev's chances to live dropped to near zero. He was septic, and his lungs were 92 percent colonized by klebsiella. "They were essentially destroyed," he says. "I had nothing left to breathe with."

At that point, a lung transplant became Zvyagintsev's only option. That also meant that his cinema career would essentially be over. Transplant recipients rarely if ever get their full verve and vigor back and must take immunosuppressants for the rest of their lives to prevent their bodies from rejecting the new organs their immune systems see as foreign. Zvyagintsev would never be able to withstand the rigorous, exhausting, long-day filming schedules.

But before the doctors could even attempt a transplant, they had to curtail the klebsiella's wrath to prevent it from colonizing Zvyagintsev's new lungs. So if antibiotics couldn't suppress it, the transplant was off the table.

At that crucial point, another one of Zvyagintsev's attending physicians uttered the word *bacteriophage*.

In an uncanny stroke of luck, Zvyagintsev's Hannover hospital had a National Center for Phage Therapy, a research institution studying the potential of living medicines. Far from an approved therapeutic modality, phages in Germany were still in an experimental state, but similar to Patterson's case, Zvyagintsev's doctors were willing to give it a try. "He was on his third week of coma and had nothing to lose," Anya says.

The Zvyagintsevs aren't sure exactly what paperwork and regulatory approvals his attending physicians followed, but because the Phage Therapy Center had a collection of phages, growing them based on Zvyagintsev's isolate took less than two days. Axel Haverich, then medical director of the MHH Clinic for Cardiac, Thoracic, Transplant, and Vascular Surgery, aggressively accelerated the process. The living medicines came back from the lab within thirty-six hours, Anya recalls. And they went to work immediately.

Zvyagintsev received his living medicines intravenously and through an inhaler—to send them directly to the infection's source. Similar to other phage treatment cases, it only took a few days for him to feel better. When his fever dropped and his breathing improved, the doctors began prepping him for the transplant, the first step for which was to take the most recent image of his wrecked lungs. And that's where the biggest surprise awaited.

Once over 90 percent destroyed, his lungs now looked completely normal. Not only was the klebsiella gone, but the damage done by it—previously deemed irreparable—was healing. The phage, initially aimed to prepare Zvyagintsev for the transplant, had done its job so well that he no longer needed a set of new lungs. The lungs he had lived with all his life repaired themselves just fine—and remarkably quickly. "The doctors who looked at my images couldn't believe it," he recalls. "They didn't think it was possible."

After spending several months in ICU and forty days in a coma, it took Zvyagintsev a long time to bounce back. The first few months after being discharged from the hospital, he lived in a wheelchair, attending a rehabilitation clinic in France. In the meantime, Russia invaded Ukraine, and Zvyagintsev and his wife decided not to return to Moscow. Yet he was healthy enough to resume cinema: in the fall of 2023, a new project was waiting for him in Paris. He and Anya fully believe that the living medicines saved his life—and career too. To keep his lungs healthy, he connected with the Eliava Institute, which now grows custom-made klebsiella-fighting phages for him. "They come in the mail, and I inhale them for prophylaxis," he says. "I should've been dead. But I am alive. And breathing with lungs that once were almost fully destroyed. It was nothing short of a miracle."[25]

PHAGES FOR GLOBAL HEALTH

The tropical sun shines brightly over a group of scientists dipping buckets into a dark sewage stream in Kenya. It's midafternoon, so the temperatures are rising along with the smell, which—in Biswajit Biswas's view—makes it a perfect moment to hunt for phages, which are happily devouring some of the worst scourges afflicting people in many African countries. All of these bucket-wielding scientists are from the African continent, and they are here to learn how to find and use living medicines for the patients fighting bacterial infectious diseases back home.

The group is partaking in a workshop organized by a nonprofit organization called Phages for Global Health. Antibiotic resistance is expected to claim ten million lives a year by 2050, but just like every other health calamity, it will unevenly affect the low- and middle-income countries, or LMIC. "We focus on LMIC because ninety percent of the deaths from antimicrobial resistance are expected to occur there," says Tobi Nagel, the organization's founder. "So we facilitate the application of phages in Africa and Asia." The idea is to empower drug development in the ways that are both biologically and culturally appropriate, she explains, by finding phages that work on the specific bacteria implicated in local outbreaks, and making phage cocktails that can be stored and transported at ambient temperatures because refrigeration is not always an option. "Look at the Covid-19 vaccines that need to be stored at minus eighty," she says. "That's not realistic for most LMIC."

There's a bigger concern too, she adds. Drug development predominantly takes place in industrialized countries. More often than not, there's a huge time gap before the medicines arrive at LMIC. And even when they do, they are often inaccessible—too expensive and in insufficient supply. "For antimicrobial resistance, that's going to result in millions of deaths," Nagel says.

Phages are cheaper and readily available alternatives. The same old Soviet wisdom makes perfect sense here. You don't need to build sophisticated factories to grow phages. You don't need expensive equipment. All your raw ingredients—the bacteria and their eaters—can be sourced from nature, right under your feet. One needs to know how to isolate phages and grow them—and that's what the workshops are for. When d'Hérelle cured plague in Egypt in 1925, the local health authority Conseil Sanitaire wrote that "India ought to arm itself."[26] That's exactly what these scientists and physicians are doing at the sewage stream: arming themselves with alternatives. "There's already about five hundred phages isolated by different researchers in Kenya," Nagel shares.

Nagel is also on the board of PhagePro, a company developing cholera phages with a long-term plan to run a clinical trial with colleagues in Bangladesh, which circles back to d'Hérelle and Eliava's time. Now we know a lot more about cholera than we did in the early 1900s, which will factor into the preparations. "Cholera is unique amongst infectious diseases in a way that the exact bacterial strains you find in one region of the world are almost identical to those that you find in another part of the world," Nagel explains. "So if we get it approved in one place, we should be able to use it and it should work in another place."

Nagel's other aim is campylobacter, a bug that commonly dwells on poultry and sickens people when they consume undercooked chicken. "We considered writing a grant with Intralytix for our campylobacter project, but we couldn't come to an agreement that could work for their company financially," she says. "If we get to the manufacturing stage, we'll see if we can get a grant together for that." Yet another is the Buruli ulcer, a neglected tropical disease rare in the Western world, but in some places in Africa, a quarter of the population can be infected.[27] Caused by *Mycobacterium ulcerans* that eats through the skin, it creates open wounds; while it still responds to antibiotics, phages may be a cheaper and easier alternative.

Nagel's path to phage therapy was, unsurprisingly, through Georgia. She had worked in big pharma and biotech start-ups for fifteen years, but she always wanted to help patients in places that had little access to the medicines she worked to bring to market. "Drug development is expensive, I know that," she says. "So I was always thinking of the more cost-effective ways to do it." She landed a consulting gig in Georgia teaching Eliava scientists about presenting and advertising their work to the rest of the world. When she understood how living medicines worked, she realized that was the solution she had been looking for. "This is a more tractable technology, it's been around for a hundred years, and it doesn't require advanced equipment." In 2016, she formed Phages for Global Health and started organizing workshops, taught by an international team of well-established phage scientists. In her recent workshop series, the PPB (Poisons and Pharmacy Board), Kenya's version of the FDA, began discussing how to put together the first compassionate use case to treat a patient with phage therapeutics.

There are also discussions about who should and how to maintain phage banks, which need to be constantly updated, just like they were in the Soviet Union. "We think the governments would have to step in and maintain these collections for the sake of public health," Nagel says. Because, she adds, the world just can't sit and wait for new antibiotics any longer. The next antibiotic-resistant blight has likely already evolved. It is just waiting for the opportune moment.[28]

We'd better have a few phages ready when it hits.

15

Phaging into the Future

In the hushed, well-lit rooms of the Eliava Institute production facility, phages are chewing through their microbial foodstuff. Growing inside large glass containers that look like supersize jars, they will be soon harvested, purified, and turned into medicines. In the adjacent room, workers are already preparing the next bacterial batch. The institute's conveyor, once nearly destroyed by politics, armed conflicts, and economic woes, is making living medicines again.

Only about fifty people work on phage production today—a fraction of what the staff used to be during the 1970s' heyday. But that's still a triumph given the history behind it. Mzia Kutateladze, the institute's current director, hopes that the worst of the economic struggles are finally behind them. "We created a nonprofit Eliava Foundation, and then the foundation created several spin-offs," she says. "We have a pharmacy. We have a clinic where patients come not only from all over Georgia but from other countries. We offer diagnostic services to them. They can buy the phages we grow here. We also offer personalized medicine service where we find and grow the specific phages they need." The profits from various spin-off companies go to the foundation to keep it afloat. "It's an American model," says Kutateladze. "And it's very unique for this part of the world."[1]

Having celebrated its centennial anniversary in 2023, the institute's manufacturing arm makes six different standard phage preparations. Manager Vakhtang Pavlenishvili gives me the inventory run-through, stacking the colorful boxes on his desk. I feel strangely nostalgic looking for my childhood friend ΦΑΓ, which started my fascination with bacteria eaters, but I can't spot the word. I realize the boxes bear no Cyrillic letters at all. With the institute's Russian days long over, the preparations' names are now written in English. Only the institute's logo—a roundish phage-like head held by thin phage-like legs—bears a fleeting semblance to the letter Φ, but even that may be a figment of my imagination. Each box boasts a different name and a different assemblage of phages on the cover. Inside there are neat little bottles with tightly closed lids, a few ounces of phage in each. They are sold in every pharmacy in Tbilisi and in many throughout Georgia.

"When my son has a sore throat, he gargles with Pyophage," Pavlenishvili says. "He really likes the taste. Actually, I don't know why, but it seems that all kids like how phages taste." Adults don't necessarily agree, he adds. "It's not a bad taste, just a different taste, and for some reason, kids like it. After he gargles, he can spit it out, but he likes to swallow it."

There's no harm in drinking Pyophage. The cocktail treats streptococcus, which causes strep and several other bugs that can cause a sore throat or infect other soft tissues. Another cocktail named Enko is formulated to extinguish the typical stomach infection culprits: shigella, salmonella, *E.coli*, and staph. The next one, Intestiphage, adds two more bacteria eaters into the mix that fight enterococcus and proteus. "When people travel someplace, they often bring a couple of boxes with them," Pavlenishvili shares. "For something like traveler's diarrhea, you may only need a dose or two. And for a serious infection, you would need a weeklong course."

Other boxes list familiar pathogen names in various combinations: SES targets staph, *E.coli,* and strep. Fersisi treats staph and strep. And then there's one that contains staph alone, boasting a yellow-orange hue on the packaging—the color of the golden devil that killed mothers and infants, closed hospitals, and evolved to evade the most potent antibiotics humans made. That same golden devil that David Shrayer-Petrov hunted in the frozen Siberian towns, sometimes with the Eliava Institute's bacteriophage on hand.

"Can this phage work against MRSA?" I ask.

"Yes, of course," Pavlenishvili answers matter-of-factly. MRSA doesn't elicit the same response in Georgians as it does in me. We fear it because MRSA learned to dodge methicillin, but for phage purposes, it's just another staph. MRSA can be deadly when you don't have options. In Georgia, this option has existed for the past fifty years. The Georgian mantra goes, "If the antibiotic doesn't work, try the phage," just like Sandro had once said in his first conversation with Glenn.

This specific staph slayer is the grandchild of the phage Teimuraz Chanishvili bred in his lab and used to save Avtandil Chkeidze and later the Moscow newborns. "This particular staph bacteriophage was formulated in the 1970s for intravenous use, so it has a more complex purification process than all other phages," Pavlenishvili tells me. "That's why this phage solution is clear while others are slightly yellow," he explains. The yellow broth is the remains of the fermentation and microbial warfare that the FDA does not want in the phage solutions. That broth is one reason why the Eliava Institute still can't take its living medicines to the international markets—it can't sell phages in Europe or the US. The other reason is the fact that the institute still doesn't have manufacturing faculties that satisfy the strict GMP rules required for medicine productions. But that's coming soon, Kutateladze tells me.

"We started to work in this direction in 2014," she says. The biggest challenge was the cost—around $2.5 million, a steep price for the still-struggling institution. "With the help of the European Union, we renovated part of our production facility and we built the so-called clean rooms, and we updated our filtration systems," she shares. "Now we have to make more clean rooms so we can prepare our initial stocks of phages in them. We are very busy with all of that, and we're hoping to finish it soon." The GMP facilities will be a game changer because they will enable the institute to finally produce and sell phages to a much wider market.

Keeping the production process clean and free of any microorganisms is key. Imagine this, Pavlenishvili says. You're aiming to grow phages against staph. You seed your broth with staph bacteria, but somehow a handful of *E.coli* flies in the door and wiggles its way into your broth. Both bacteria happily grow. Then you inoculate the brew with staph phages that wipe out only the staph bacteria while *E.coli* proliferates unrestrained. Now your phage preparation is garbage, and you must start anew. The GMP facilities assure that this doesn't happen.[2]

While the GMP facilities are being built, the institute is shipping phages for agricultural use to some European collaborators for the same reason Intralytix chose to pursue the food industry first: the regulations are far less stringent. As European farmers curtail antibiotic use, they need an alternative to keep animals healthy. In some European countries, phages are considered natural products, which normally dwell in cowsheds and pigsties—basically a form of probiotics. So adding some more phages that specifically go after certain unwanted pathogenic organisms doesn't require complicated approval hurdles. "In Germany, for example, farmers are free to use phages if they want," Pavlenishvili says. "Because these are the natural products, made from phages found in nature, and not genetically modified, farmers can use them."

The phage-making team monitors bacterial evolution closely in order to keep their phage library up-to-date at all times. "We collect data about our phage efficiency every day," says Pavlenishvili. "And then, every six months, people sit down and look at this data. For example, if in January our staph bacteriophage was ninety-five percent effective against *Staphylococcus aureus* and in June it is ninety-four percent effective, that's okay, we don't have to do anything. But if it went down to seventy or fifty percent, that is an indication that we have to do something. We either have to retrain this phage or use another one from our collection. That's a continuous process."

"What happens if you don't have a phage that works?" I ask.

Pavlenishvili shrugs, just as matter-of-factly as he did with my MRSA question. "We just go back to the river," he says. To Mtkvari, whose good waters started it all more than one hundred years ago. It will never run out of phages.

The next day, Nina Chanishvili takes me over to the French cottage built by Eliava for his and d'Hérelle's family. The cottage is still there and so is the green iron fence that surrounds it, so tall one can barely see the building itself. "Not a soul knows what's inside or who it belongs to," Nina tells me. "After all these years, it's still a mystery." I try to see above the fence, but the trees on the inside block the view. There's no sign and no plaque, but the building is in good shape—in fact, it's in better shape than the one Nina's laboratory is in. Somebody is taking care of it. "We walk by it all the time, and we don't have the slightest idea who owns it," Nina keeps talking. "To this day, it remains a secret."

Later, my Tbilisi tour guide Margo Gelovani and I try to find the apartment building where Eliava's family lived when he was arrested. After searching several blocks in the city center, we think we finally found it. I take a few pictures of the façade. When I show them to Natalia Devdariani-Malieva, she tells me that's the wrong house. The original building has long been demolished, she says. A century later, there's little left. Except for phages and the institute now proudly bearing Eliava's name.

Eliava and d'Hérelle envisioned the institute as an international bacteriophage research hub. Their vision never fully materialized because of corruption, politics, dictatorships, and greed. But in a way, their brainchild has accomplished much more. For about one hundred years now, it served as a time capsule, preserving the knowledge accumulated and written down by its founders. Today, much of the phage identification, growth, and purification methods still date back to d'Hérelle's original techniques outlined in his monographs, including his last one, written in Tbilisi and translated by Eliava. Sometimes referred to as the "phage bible," *The Bacteriophage and the Phenomenon of Recovery* raised generations of phage-keepers who held on to that wisdom.

These phage-keepers were tenacious. They preserved their knowledge despite all odds. They stashed their living medicines in their home refrigerators. They showed up in the lab even when they had not been paid for months. They sat through work meetings in winter coats. Sandro spent countless days arguing with naysayers and numerous late nights wondering how to pay Intralytix's bills without going under. One day, when Mzia Kutateladze and Steffanie Strathdee met in person, they talked about how hard it was to get the world to listen. "I told Mzia I felt really embarrassed that they have been working on this for decades and they have so much experience, and it's some American who gets phage therapy and all of a sudden the West wakes up," Steffanie recalls.[3]

"Yes, it's hard sometimes," Mzia answered. "We've being working on disseminating and offering this knowledge, and for so many years, we've been getting nowhere." She's hopeful that's finally changing.[4]

Sandro hopes so too. Tom Patterson's case might have been the perfect storm, but that storm fell onto fertile soil, which he had been cultivating for over two decades. Today, Intralytix is the only American bacteriophage company that remained operational since its launch in 1998. While others came and went, Intralytix has operated continuously for a quarter of a century, celebrating its twenty-five-year anniversary in June 2023, coinciding with the Eliava Institute's centennial. "I don't know if I would have started it if I knew how difficult it would be," Sandro says, reflecting on his long journey. "Well, I probably would've anyway. Every time I considered quitting, I thought of Glenn's patient who died from VRE and the fact that he could've been saved—as well as hundreds of other people."

People told him to quit. They said the idea was hopeless. They had many very logical reasons, Sandro recalls. "I was told that the FDA will never approve a phage product for either food safety or therapeutic use. But they did. Then I was told that the FDA will never approve a phage cocktail with multiple viruses in it, because it's too many variables. But they did. And finally, I was told that the FDA will never consider a clinical trial in which we would treat people with a live virus. And, look, they have approved it too. That's not a coincidence. For years, we've been showing the FDA that we know how to do it. And we proved, one spray at a time, that phages were safe." And by doing that, Intralytix laid the foundation for others.

"He's a very admirable early warrior in the phage space," says Paul Garofolo, the CEO of Locus Biosciences. Developing phage food sprays helped legitimize phage therapeutic applications for many other companies who came after him. The food safety sprays that Intralytix developed eventually afforded phages the coveted description of "generally recognized as safe," or GRAS, says Garofolo. "That helped create some GRAS designations for certain agricultural products and helped build awareness of the safety profile," he says.[5] Two decades down the road, the phages were no longer scary, unfamiliar entities with a dark "commie science" history. They have proven themselves as humanity's potent allies that could save lives when used properly.

Sandro was also prescient in his assessment of the lytic phages (which burst bacteria) versus the temperate ones (that hide in the bacteria genome). He thought the concern was overblown, and he was right. Scientists have found that temperate phages can become non-temperate or lytic killers, but the opposite doesn't happen. Lytic phages don't change their modus operandi. Essentially once a phage is a killer, it's always a killer. "People have made temperate phages into non-temperate phages," says E. Scott Stibitz, a colleague of Cara Fiore, who leads a phage lab at the FDA's CBER department, "but it is virtually impossible to turn a lytic phage into a temperate phage; they are completely different."[6]

Similarly, modern technology can now put another concern to rest: phages accidently transferring toxic genes into a relatively harmless bacteria and making it a monster. Twenty-five years ago, when Sandro formed Intralytix, it wasn't possible to sequence every phage. Now the sequencing technology is affordable and widely available, so every phage and every gene can be described and cataloged. Several research institutions have projects dedicated to sequencing and cataloging phages so no future phage therapeutics will harbor scary surprises.

Some challenges still remain. Phages are the only medicines that multiply as they work. That still presents a dosage conundrum. Exactly how does one figure out a proper dose? Moreover, different phages make different amounts of progeny. Some produce only ten copies inside the bacteria they invade, while others can make a hundred or more. But what's clear is that humanity found a formidable ally against the never-ending bacterial threat—and we have finally figured out how to engage with it properly.

Louis Pasteur once said that the microbes will have the last word. And for a good reason. The microbes have millions of years of tricks they can use against us. On the evolutionary scale, we humans are too young and inexperienced a species to fight against them. We can't outsmart, outwit, or outbid the innumerable variety of nimble microscopic organisms with fluid genes and enormous capacities to reshuffle them quickly. But we can sic them on each other, take a back seat, and watch the battle. Louis Pasteur was right. The microbes will indeed have the last word. But some of them—such as the ΦΑΓ I painted in rainbow colors as a child—may tip the scales in our favor.

ACKNOWLEDGMENTS

No woman is an island. No author can write a book on their own. I am no exception. This book would not have happened, had it not been for the many wonderfully forthcoming people who so graciously welcomed me into their homes, their laboratories, and their lives. This book would not have happened had they not showed me their work, their research, and their family pictures. This book would not have happened had they not sat down with me around their dinner tables, sharing their meals and memories with me late into the night.

I owe my endless thanks to Nina Chanishvili, who spent two weeks taking me through the Eliava Institute's hundred years' worth of history, unearthing handwritten notes of coworkers long gone, decades-old newspaper clips in Russian and Georgian, and translating early phage studies from French to English for me. And for presenting me with a surprise birthday cake, along the way.

I am eternally grateful to Natalia Devdariani-Malieva for sharing with me her tragic family history and her mother's memoir—as well as for teaching me to crack the Easter eggs the Georgian way. I'm also grateful to her son, Dimitry Devdariani. Without their stories I would not have been able to bring Giorgi Eliava, his wife Amelia, and their daughter Ganna to life.

I thank Timothy Blauvelt for sharing the documents he obtained from the Georgian KGB archives, without which I would not have pieced together the terror and injustice suffered by my characters.

I thank Dmitriy Myelnikov for sharing his research on the Soviet era phage use.

I thank Mzia Kutateladze for her insights into the Eliava Institute's past and present.

I thank Maxim Shrayer, the son of David Shrayer-Petrov, for sharing his father's books and papers with me, which were invaluable for constructing the scenes of devastation caused by *Staphylococcus aureus* in Soviet Siberia and Félix d'Hérelle's experience in Russia.

I thank William Summers for his insights into Félix d'Hérelle's biography. I thank Steffanie Strathdee for connecting me with Graham Hatfull and Carl Merril, who, in turn, connected me with Biswajit Biswas.

I thank Robert "Chip" Schooley for finding time to read over my descriptions of antibiotic-resistant dysentery and confirm I've got it right.

I will always be thankful to Sandro's cousins Natela, Maia, and Mikhail Okudjava for a wonderful night of family memories that helped me recreate his childhood world.

I am grateful to Sandro Sulakvelidze, who put up with my intermittent barrage of emails, Zooms, visits, and pleas for fact-checking for the four years I spent working on this book.

Finally, I would like to thank the people who worked with me to bring this book into the world. I thank my agent, Luba Ostashevsky, who thought my seed of an idea could become a narrative. I thank my editor, George Witte, for guiding me through the process and for his insightful comments that made this book the best it could be. Lastly, I thank Brigitte Dale for shepherding my manuscript through its many milestones. Thank you all for taking *The Living Medicine* to the finish line. I would not have done it without you.

NOTES

1. The Surge of the Superbugs

1. Tyson J. Ruetz, Ann E. Lin, and Julian A. Guttman, "*Shigella flexneri* Utilize the Spectrin Cytoskeleton during Invasion and Comet Tail Generation," *BMC Microbiology*, March 16, 2012, https://doi.org/10.1186/1471-2180-12-36.

2. "Shigella: Diagnosis and Treatment," Centers for Disease Control and Prevention, last reviewed April 6, 2023, https://www.cdc.gov/shigella/diagnosistreatment.html.

3. Kim Krieger, "Discovering What Makes This Toxin Even Worse Than Diarrhea," UConn Today, January 6, 2021, https://today.uconn.edu/2021/01/discovering-makes-toxin-even-worse-diarrhea/#.

4. "Increase in Extensively Drug-Resistant Shigellosis in the United States," Centers for Disease Control and Prevention, February 24, 2023, https://emergency.cdc.gov/han/2023/han00486.asp.

5. "Epidemiology, Testing, and Management of Extensively Drug-Resistant Shigellosis," Centers for Disease Control and Prevention, February 28, 2023, https://emergency.cdc.gov/coca/calls/2023/callinfo_022823.asp.

6. "More People in the United States Dying from Antibiotic-Resistant Infections than Previously Estimated," Centers for Disease Control and Prevention, November 13, 2019, https://archive.cdc.gov/www_cdc_gov/media/releases/2019/p1113-antibiotic-resistant.html.

7. Sandro Sulakvelidze, interview with the author, February 28, 2023.

8. "Staph Infections Can Kill," *CDC Vital Signs*, March 5, 2019, https://www.cdc.gov/vitalsigns/staph/pdf/vs-0305-staph-infections-h.pdf.

9. WebMD Editorial Contributors, "What Is VRE?," WebMD, September 18, 2023, https://www.webmd.com/skin-problems-and-treatments/what-is-vre.

10. *Antibiotic Resistance Threats in the United States, 2019* (Atlanta, GA: CDC, 2019), https://www.cdc.gov/drugresistance/pdf/threats-report/2019-ar-threats-report-508.pdf.

11. Christopher JI Murray et al., "Global Burden of Bacterial Antimicrobial Resistance in 2019: A Systematic Analysis," *The Lancet,* February 12, 2022, https://doi.org/10.1016/S0140-6736(21)02724-0.

12. *COVID-19: U.S. Impact on Antimicrobial Resistance, 2022 Special Report* (Atlanta, GA: US Department of Health and Human Services, 2022), 3, https://www.cdc.gov/drugresistance/covid19.html.

13. "UN, Global Health Agencies Sound Alarm on Drug-Resistant Infections; New Recommendations to Reduce 'Staggering Number' of Future Deaths," *UN News,* April 29, 2019, https://news.un.org/en/story/2019/04/1037471.

14. "Frequently Asked Questions (FAQ) About Plague," Centers for Disease Control and Prevention, last reviewed April 4, 2018, https://emergency.cdc.gov/agent/plague/faq.asp#.

15. "NIH Awards Grants to Support Bacteriophage Therapy Research," National Institutes of Health, March 11, 2021, https://www.nih.gov/news-events/news-releases/nih-awards-grants-support-bacteriophage-therapy-research.

16. Sulakvelidze interview, February 28, 2023.

17. "Estimates of Foodborne Illness in the United States," Centers for Disease Control and Prevention, last reviewed November 5, 2018, https://www.cdc.gov/foodborneburden/index.html.

18. Sulakvelidze interview, February 28, 2023.

19. Natela, Maia, and Mikhail Okudjava (Sandro's cousins), interview with the author, April 22, 2022.

20. Natela, Maia, and Mikhail Okudjava interview. April 22, 2022.

21. Sulakvelidze interview, January 17, 2022.

22. Sulakvelidze interview, September 30, 2022.

23. Sulakvelidze interview, September 30, 2022.

24. Sulakvelidze interview, September 30, 2022.

25. Nina Chanishvili, interview with the author, April 18, 2023.

26. Sulakvelidze interview, September 30, 2022.

27. Sulakvelidze interview, September 30, 2022.

28. Sulakvelidze interview, September 30, 2022.

29. Sulakvelidze interview, September 30, 2022.

30. Alexander Sulakvelidze et al., "Production of Enterotoxin by *Yersinia bercovieri,* a Recently Identified *Yersinia enterocolitica*–Like Species," *Infection and Immunity* 67, no. 2 (1999), https://doi.org/10.1128/iai.67.2.968-971.1999.

31. Glenn Morris, interview with the author, December 20, 2021.
32. Morris interview, December 20, 2021.

2. The Parasite of Microbes

1. Miriam Reid, "John Snow Hunts the Blue Death," *Distillations Magazine*, Science History Institute, March 8, 2022, https://www.sciencehistory.org/distillations/john-snow-hunts-the-blue-death.

2. Irakli Georgadze, *Materiali Ubileinogo Simposiuma* [Materials for the anniversary symposium] (Tbilisi, Georgia: Science Research Center for Vaccines and Serums, 1974), 8.

3. *Report about the Work of the Georgian Central Bacteriological Laboratory*, 1921, handwritten notes, 1, Eliava Institute archives, Tbilisi, Georgia.

4. Eliava-Malieva, memoir, *Russian Club* magazine, April 2017, part X, 32.

5. Margo Gelovani (Tbilisi tour and history guide), interview with the author, April 22, 2022.

6. Eliava-Malieva, memoir, unedited version, Devdariani-Malieva family archives, 13.

7. Natalia Devdariani-Malieva (granddaughter of Giorgi Eliava), interview with the author, April 18, 2022.

8. Anna Kuchment, *The Forgotten Cure: The Past and Future of Phage Therapy* (New York: Springer, 2012), 25.

9. Nina Chanishvili, Dmitriy Myelnikov, and Timothy K. Blauvelt, "Professor Giorgi Eliava and the Eliava Institute of Bacteriophage," *Phage* 3, no. 2 (2022), figure 2, https://doi.org/10.1089/phage.2022.0016. "Georges Eliava" is listed as enrolled student #206.

10. "Cristiani, Hector," Swiss Elite Database, https://www2.unil.ch/elitessuisses/personne.php?id=75589.

11. "Cholera," Institut Pasteur, https://www.pasteur.fr/en/medical-center/disease-sheets/cholera.

12. Gelovani interview, April 22, 2022.

13. Gelovani interview, April 22, 2022.

14. Félix d'Hérelle, *Bacteriophage: Its Role in Immunity*, trans. George Smith (Baltimore: William & Wilkins, 1922), 18.

15. Félix d'Hérelle, *Bacteriophage and the Phenomenon of Recovery* [in Russian], trans. Giorgi Eliava (Georgia: Tiflis State University Publishing, 1935), 12.

16. William C. Summers, *Félix d'Hérelle and the Origins of Molecular Biology* (New Haven, CT: Yale University Press, 1999), 48.

17. William C. Summers, "In the Beginning," *Bacteriophage* 1, no. 1 (2011): 50–1, https://doi.org/10.4161/bact.1.1.14070.

18. Alain Dublanchet and Shawna Bourne, "The Epic of Phage Therapy," *Canadian Journal of Infectious Diseases and Medical Microbiology* 18, no. 1 (2007): 15–8, https://doi.org/10.1155/2007/365761.

19. Dublanchet and Bourne, "Epic of Phage Therapy."

20. Summers, "In the Beginning."

21. Dublanchet and Bourne, "Epic of Phage Therapy."

22. Hervé Lecoq, "Discovery of the First Virus, Tobacco Mosaic Virus: 1892 or 1898?," *Comptes Rendus de l'Académie des Sciences-Series III-Sciences de la Vie* 324, no. 10 (2001): 929–33, https://doi .org/10.1016/s0764-4469(01)01368-3.

23. David Shrayer-Petrov, *Félix d'Hérelle in Russia* (Providence, RI: Roger Williams Medical Center, 1996), 1; David Shrayer-Petrov, "Félix d'Hérelle in Russia," *Bulletin de l'Institut Pasteur* 94 (1996): 91–6.

24. Félix d'Hérelle, "On an Invisible Microbe Antagonistic Toward Dysenteric Bacilli: Brief Note by Mr. F. d'Herelle," 1917, https://doi .org/10.1016/j.resmic.2007.07.005, digitized in 2007.

25. Summers, *Félix d'Hérelle*, 4.

26. Summers, *Félix d'Hérelle*, 192.

27. Eliava-Malieva, memoir, part III.

28. Devdariani-Malieva interview, April 18, 2022

29. Devdariani-Malieva interview, April 18, 2022.

30. Kuchment, *The Forgotten Cure*, 26.

31. Eliava-Malieva, memoir, part V.

3. A Georgian in Paris

1. William C. Summers, "In the Beginning," *Bacteriophage* 1, no. 1 (2011): 50–1, https://doi.org/10.4161/bact.1.1.14070.

2. "Jules Bordet," Nobel Prizes and Laureats, https://www.nobelprize .org/prizes/medicine/1919/bordet/facts/.

3. Ernest Hankin, "The Bactericidal Action of the Waters of the Jamuna and Ganges Rivers on Cholera Microbes," Ann. Inst. Pasteur 10:511–523 (1896), *Bacteriophage* 1, no. 3 (2011): 117–26, https: //doi.org/10.4161/bact.1.3.16736.

4. Félix d'Hérelle, *Bacteriophage and the Phenomenon of Recovery* [in Russian], trans. Giorgi Eliava (Georgia: Tiflis State University Publishing, 1935), 11–2.

5. Summers, "In the Beginning."

6. Alain Dublanchet and Shawna Bourne, "The Epic of Phage Therapy," *Canadian Journal of Infectious Diseases and Medical Microbiology* 18, no. 1 (2007): 15–8, https://doi.org/10.1155/2007/365761.

7. Dublanchet and Bourne, "Epic of Phage Therapy."

8. Dublanchet and Bourne, "Epic of Phage Therapy."

9. Dublanchet and Bourne, "Epic of Phage Therapy."

10. Lyudmila Scherbina-Esvangia, "Georgia Needs Me!," *Zarya Vostoka*, June 23, 1988.

11. Natalia Devdariani-Malieva (granddaughter of Giorgi Eliava), interview with the author, April 18, 2022.

12. Scherbina-Esvangia, "Georgia Needs Me!"

13. Scherbina-Esvangia, "Georgia Needs Me!"

14. Devdariani-Malieva interview, April 18, 2022.

15. Devdariani-Malieva interview, April 18, 2022.

16. Anna Kuchment, *The Forgotten Cure: The Past and Future of Phage Therapy* (New York: Springer, 2012), 11.

17. Félix d'Hérelle, *Bacteriophage: Its Role in Immunity*, trans. George Smith (Baltimore: William & Wilkins, 1922), 264.

18. Alexander Sulakvelidze and Elizabeth Kutter, eds., *Bacteriophages: Biology and Applications* (Boca Raton, FL: CRC Press, 2004), 383.

19. Kuchment, *The Forgotten Cure*, 11.

20. Sulakvelidze and Kutter, *Bacteriophages*, 383.

21. D'Hérelle, *Bacteriophage: Its Role in Immunity*, 264.

22. William C. Summers, *Félix d'Hérelle and the Origins of Molecular Biology* (New Haven, CT: Yale University Press, 1999), 114–5.

23. Summers, *Félix d'Hérelle*, 117–8.

24. Chika N. Okafor, Ayesan Rewane, and Ifeanyi I. Momodu, "Bacillus Calmette Guerin," StatPearls [Internet], last updated July 3, 2023, https://www.ncbi.nlm.nih.gov/books/NBK538185/.

25. Summers, *Félix d'Hérelle*, 66–7, quoting d'Hérelle's memoir.

26. Summers, *Félix d'Hérelle*, quoting d'Hérelle's memoir.

27. D'Hérelle, *Bacteriophage: Its Role in Immunity*, 61–3.

28. D'Hérelle, *Bacteriophage: Its Role in Immunity*, 61–3.

29. D'Hérelle, *Bacteriophage: Its Role in Immunity*, 61–3.

30. D'Hérelle, *Bacteriophage: Its Role in Immunity*, 61–3.

31. D'Hérelle, *Bacteriophage: Its Role in Immunity*, 61–3.

32. D'Hérelle, *Bacteriophage: Its Role in Immunity*, 149.

33. "Staph Infections Can Kill," *CDC Vital Signs*, March 5, 2019, https://www.cdc.gov/vitalsigns/staph/pdf/vs-0305-staph-infections-h.pdf.

34. D'Hérelle, *Bacteriophage: Its Role in Immunity*, 98.

35. Ganna Eliava-Malieva, memoir, *Russian Club* magazine, March 2017, part VI, 33.

36. Eliava-Malieva, memoir, part VI, 34.

37. Eliava-Malieva, memoir, part VI, 34.

38. Eliava-Malieva, memoir, part VI, 34.

39. Eliava-Malieva, memoir, part VI, 34; Devdariani-Malieva interview, April 18, 2022.

40. Eliava-Malieva, memoir, part VI, 34.

4. Phages Rise to Fame and Glory

1. Natalia Devdariani-Malieva (granddaughter of Giorgi Eliava), interview with the author, April 18, 2022.

2. Irakli Georgadze, *Materiali Ubileinogo Simposiuma* [Materials for the anniversary symposium] (Tbilisi, Georgia: Science Research Center for Vaccines and Serums, 1974), 10–1.

3. Georgadze, *Materiali Ubileinogo Simposiuma*, 11–12.

4. Georgadze, *Materiali Ubileinogo Simposiuma*, 13.

5. Georgadze, *Materiali Ubileinogo Simposiuma*, 13.

6. Ganna Eliava-Malieva, memoir, *Russian Club* magazine, March 2017.

7. William C. Summers, *Félix d'Hérelle and the Origins of Molecular Biology* (New Haven, CT: Yale University Press, 1999), 125–6.

8. Summers, *Félix d'Hérelle*, 125–6.

9. Summers, *Félix d'Hérelle*, 125–6.

10. Thomas Häusler, *Viruses vs. Superbugs: A Solution to the Antibiotic Crisis?* (London: Palgrave Macmillan, 2006), 80–1.

11. Summers, *Félix d'Hérelle*, 126.

12. Summers, *Félix d'Hérelle*, 126.

13. Summers, *Félix d'Hérelle*, 118.

14. Summers, *Félix d'Hérelle*, 118.

15. Félix d'Hérelle, *Bacteriophage and the Phenomenon of Recovery* [in

Russian], trans. Giorgi Eliava (Georgia: Tiflis State University Publishing, 1935), 169.

16. Félix d'Hérelle, *Les defenses de l'organisme* (Paris: Flammarion, 1923), https://www.worldcat.org/title/defenses-de-lorganisme/oclc /11127665.

17. Summers, *Félix d'Hérelle*, 118–9.

18. Summers, *Félix d'Hérelle*, 122.

19. Summers, *Félix d'Hérelle*, 128.

20. Summers, *Félix d'Hérelle*, 128.

21. Summers, *Félix d'Hérelle*, 128.

22. G. Eliava, *"Au sejet de l'adsorption du bacteriophage par les leucocytes"* [On the subject of bacteriophage adsorption by leukocytes], *Comptes Rendus des Seances de la Societe de Biologie et de Ses Filiales* 105 (1930): 829–31, translated for the author from French by Nina Chanishvili.

23. Eliava, *"Au sejet de l'adsorption."*

24. Eliava, *"Au sejet de l'adsorption."*

25. G. Eliava and E. Suarez, "Dimensions of the Bacteriophage Carpuscle" [in French], *Comptes Rendus des Seances de la Societe de Biologie et de Ses Filiales* 96, no. 1 (1927): 460–2, translated for the author from French by Nina Chanishvili.

26. Gene Mayer, "Microbiology and Immunology Online," Bacteriophage, https://www.microbiologybook.org/mayer/phage.htm.

27. L. Nattan-Larrier, G. Eliava, and L. Richard, *"Bactériophage et perméabilité placentaire"* [Bacteriophage and placental permeability], *Comptes Rendus des Seances de la Societe de Biologie et de Ses Filiales* 106 (1931): 794–7, translated for the author from French by Nina Chanishvili.

28. Nina Chanishvili, Dmitriy Myelnikov, and Timothy K. Blauvelt, "Professor Giorgi Eliava and the Eliava Institute of Bacteriophage," *Phage* 3, no. 2 (2022), https://doi.org/10.1089/phage.2022.0016.

29. Chanishvili, Myelnikov, and Blauvelt, "Professor Giorgi Eliava," 74.

30. Records of Giorgi Eliava's NKVD case, scan10016.tif, Archive of the former Georgian KGB, now referred to formally as *Sakartvelos Shinagan Sakmeta Saministro (shss) arkivi (I)* [Section I of the Archive of the Ministry of Internal Affairs of Georgia], Tbilisi, Georgia.

31. Chanishvili, Myelnikov, and Blauvelt, "Professor Giorgi Eliava," 75.

32. George H. Smith, letter dated March 11, 1925, cited by William

Summers, "On the Origins of the Science in *Arrowsmith*," *Journal of the History of Medicine and Allied Sciences* 46, no. 3 (1991): 315–32, https://doi.org/10.1093/jhmas/46.3.315.

33. Summers, "On the Origins of the Science in *Arrowsmith*," cited in Anna Kuchment, *The Forgotten Cure: The Past and Future of Phage Therapy* (New York: Springer, 2012), 18.

34. "Tiny and Deadly Bacillus Has Enemies Still Smaller," *New York Times*, September 27, 1925, https://www.nytimes.com/1925/09/27/archives/tiny-and-deadly-bacillus-has-enemies-still-smaller.html.

35. "Tiny and Deadly Bacillus."

36. N. W. Larkum, "Bacteriophage from a Public Health Standpoint," *American Journal of Public Health* 19, no. 1 (1929): 31–6, https://ajph.aphapublications.org/doi/10.2105/AJPH.19.1.31.

37. Steven J. Peitzman, "Félix d'Hérelle and Bacteriophage Therapy," in *Transactions and Studies of the Philadelphia College of Physicians* (Baltimore: Waverly Press, 1970), 115–21, https://ia600901.us.archive.org/8/items/transactionsstud4371coll/transactionsstud4371coll.pdf.

38. Carl R. Merril, Dean Scholl, and Sankar L. Adhya, "The Prospect for Bacteriophage Therapy in Western Medicine," *Nature Reviews Drug Discovery* 2, no. 6 (2003): 489–97, https://doi.org/10.1038/nrd1111.

39. Häusler, *Viruses vs. Superbugs*, 92.

40. Peitzman, "Félix d'Hérelle."

41. Summers, *Félix d'Hérelle*, 163.

42. Peitzman, "Félix d'Hérelle."

43. M. P. Ravenel, "The Bacteriophage and Its Behavior," *American Journal of Public Health* 16, no. 9 (1926): 931, https://www.ncbi.nlm.nih.gov/pmc/articles/PMC1321385/.

44. Summers, *Félix d'Hérelle*, 147.

45. Summers, *Félix d'Hérelle*, 159.

5. Together in Tiflis

1. Natalia Devdariani-Malieva (granddaughter of Giorgi Eliava), interview with the author, April 18, 2022.

2. Records of Giorgi Eliava's NKVD case, Archive of the former Georgian KGB, now referred to formally as *Sakartvelos Shinagan Sakmeta Saministro (shss) arkivi (I)* [Section I of the Archive of the Ministry of Internal Affairs of Georgia], Tbilisi, Georgia.

3. Eliava's memo "*Dokladnaya Zapiska*," dated November 1932, trans-

lated from Georgian by Nina Chanishvili, Eliava Institute archives, Tbilisi, Georgia.

4. Timothy Blauvelt, "Between Modernity and Neo-Tradition: Patronage Politics and Bacteriophage Research in Interwar Soviet Georgia," *Euxeinos: Governance and Culture in the Black Sea Region* 11, no. 34 (2022): 90–114, https://doi.org/10.55337/QFSS5487.

5. Blauvelt, "Between Modernity and Neo-Tradition."

6. Blauvelt, "Between Modernity and Neo-Tradition."

7. Blauvelt, "Between Modernity and Neo-Tradition."

8. Blauvelt, "Between Modernity and Neo-Tradition."

9. William C. Summers, *Félix d'Hérelle and the Origins of Molecular Biology* (New Haven, CT: Yale University Press, 1999), 163.

10. David Shrayer-Petrov, *Félix d'Hérelle in Russia* (Providence, RI: Roger Williams Medical Center, 1996); David Shrayer-Petrov, "Félix d'Hérelle in Russia," *Bulletin de l'Institut Pasteur* 94 (1996): 91–6.

11. Alexander Sulakvelidze, Glenn Morris, and Zemphira Alavidze, "Bacteriophage Therapy," *Antimicrobial Agents and Chemotherapy* 45, no. 3 (March 2001): 649–59, https://doi.org/10.1128/aac.45.3.649-659.2001.

12. Shrayer-Petrov, *Félix d'Hérelle in Russia*; Shrayer-Petrov, "Félix d'Hérelle in Russia."

13. Blauvelt, "Between Modernity and Neo-Tradition."

14. Irakli Georgadze, *Materiali Ubileinogo Simposiuma* [Materials for the anniversary symposium] (Tbilisi, Georgia: Science Research Center for Vaccines and Serums, 1974), 22–3.

15. Félix d'Hérelle, *Bacteriophage and the Phenomenon of Recovery* [in Russian], trans. Giorgi Eliava (Georgia: Tiflis State University Publishing, 1935), 19.

16. D'Hérelle, *Bacteriophage and the Phenomenon of Recovery*, 122.

17. Shrayer-Petrov, *Félix d'Hérelle in Russia*; Shrayer-Petrov, "Félix d'Hérelle in Russia."

18. Summers, *Félix d'Hérelle*, 163.

19. Summers, *Félix d'Hérelle*, 163.

20. Georgadze, *Materiali Ubileinogo Simposiuma*, 22–3.

21. Shrayer-Petrov, *Félix d'Hérelle in Russia*; Shrayer-Petrov, "Félix d'Hérelle in Russia."

22. Dimitry Devdariani (great-grandson of Giorgi Eliava), interview with the author, April 5, 2023.

23. Nina Chanishvili, interview with the author, April 18, 2023, as told by Nunu Gelasonidze and written down by Chanishvili.

24. D'Hérelle, *Bacteriophage and the Phenomenon of Recovery*, 8–9.

25. Blauvelt, "Between Modernity and Neo-Tradition."

26. Timothy Blauvelt, interview with the author, April 22, 2023.

27. Blauvelt, "Between Modernity and Neo-Tradition."

28. Blauvelt, "Between Modernity and Neo-Tradition."

29. Blauvelt, "Between Modernity and Neo-Tradition."

30. Anna Kuchment, *The Forgotten Cure: The Past and Future of Phage Therapy* (New York: Springer, 2012), 29, citing diary of Marie and Félix d'Hérelle.

31. Natalia Devdariani-Malieva (granddaughter of Giorgi Eliava), interview with the author, April 18, 2022.

32. Blauvelt, "Between Modernity and Neo-Tradition."

33. Nina Chanishvili, Dmitriy Myelnikov, and Timothy K. Blauvelt, "Professor Giorgi Eliava and the Eliava Institute of Bacteriophage," *Phage* 3, no. 2 (2022), https://doi.org/10.1089/phage.2022.0016.

34. Chanishvili, Myelnikov, and Blauvelt, "Professor Giorgi Eliava."

35. Blauvelt, "Between Modernity and Neo-Tradition."

36. David Shrayer-Petrov, *Okhota na Ryzhevo Diavola* [Hunting down the golden devil] (Moscow: Agraf, 2010), 134.

37. Kuchment, *The Forgotten Cure*, 28, citing diary of Marie and Félix d'Hérelle.

38. Dmitriy Myelnikov, "An Alternative Cure: The Adoption and Survival of Bacteriophage Therapy in the USSR, 1922–1955," *Journal of the History of Medicine and Allied Sciences* 73, no. 4 (2018): 385–411, https://doi.org/10.1093/jhmas/jry024, citing *Pravda* 298, no. 6184, October 28, 1934, 6. On d'Hérelle's visits to Georgia, see Shrayer-Petrov, "Félix d'Hérelle in Russia"; Summers, *Félix d'Hérelle*, 161–72; Félix d'Hérelle, *Autobiographie de Félix d'Hérelle: Les Peregrinations d'un bacteriologiste*, ed. Alain Dublanchet (Paris: Editions Medicales Internationales, 2017), 311–3.

39. Myelnikov, "An Alternative Cure."

40. Myelnikov, "An Alternative Cure."

41. Summers, *Félix d'Hérelle*, 148.

42. D'Hérelle, *Bacteriophage and the Phenomenon of Recovery*, 175–7.

43. D'Hérelle, *Bacteriophage and the Phenomenon of Recovery*, 184–8.

44. D'Hérelle, *Bacteriophage and the Phenomenon of Recovery*, 184.
45. Natalia Devdariani-Malieva (granddaughter of Giorgi Eliava), interview with the author, April 18, 2022.
46. D'Hérelle, *Bacteriophage and the Phenomenon of Recovery*, preface.
47. Shrayer-Petrov, *Félix d'Hérelle in Russia*,1; Shrayer-Petrov, "Félix d'Hérelle in Russia," 5.
48. Chanishvili, Myelnikov, and Blauvelt, "Professor Giorgi Eliava."
49. Devdariani-Malieva interview with the author, April 18, 2022.

6. The Great Terror

1. Ganna Eliava-Malieva, memoir, *Russian Club* magazine, April 2017, part XII.
2. Eliava-Malieva, memoir, part XII.
3. Timothy Blauvelt, "Between Modernity and Neo-Tradition: Patronage Politics and Bacteriophage Research in Interwar Soviet Georgia," *Euxeinos: Governance and Culture in the Black Sea Region* 11, no. 34 (2022): 90–114. A law passed on December 1, 1934, in the wake of the assassination of Sergei Kirov simplified the procedure for arrest and conviction in cases of "terrorism," allowing for an in camera hearing without defense council and immediate implementation of the death penalty with no appeal. In 1937, the simplified procedure was extended to all political crimes of "wrecking" and "sabotage." See Peter H. Solomon Jr., *Soviet Criminal Justice Under Stalin* (New York: Cambridge University Press, 1996), 236–7.
4. Eliava-Malieva, memoir, part XII.
5. Nina Chanishvili, interview with the author, April 15, 2022.
6. Chanishvili interview, April 15, 2022, as told by Nunu Gelasonidze and written down by Chanishvili.
7. Natalia Devdariani-Malieva (granddaughter of Giorgi Eliava), interview with the author, April 18, 2022.
8. Devdariani-Malieva interview, April 18, 2022.
9. Eliava-Malieva, memoir, part XII.
10. Eliava-Malieva, memoir, parts XII and XIII.
11. Records of Giorgi Eliava's NKVD case, scan10087.tif, Archive of the former Georgian KGB, now referred to formally as *Sakartvelos Shinagan Sakmeta Saministro (shss) arkivi (I)* [Section I of the Archive of the Ministry of Internal Affairs of Georgia], Tbilisi, Georgia.

12. Eliava-Malieva, memoir, part X.

13. Eliava-Malieva, memoir, part XVI, 41.

14. Eliava-Malieva, memoir, part XIV.

15. Records of Eliava's NKVD case, scan10087.tif.

16. Records of Eliava's NKVD case, scan10088.tif.

17. Records of Eliava's NKVD case, scan10088.tif and scan10093.tif.

18. Blauvelt, "Between Modernity and Neo-Tradition."

19. Eliava-Malieva, memoir, part XVI, 41.

20. Devdariani-Malieva interview, April 18, 2022.

21. Eliava-Malieva, memoir, part XVI, 41.

22. Blauvelt, "Between Modernity and Neo-Tradition."

23. Eliava-Malieva, memoir, April 2017.

24. *Report About the Syphilis Treatment*, handwritten notes, not dated, scan IMG_9837.pdf, Eliava Institute archives, Tbilisi, Georgia.

7. Hell on Earth, Cholera in Water, Phages Underground

1. Zinaida Ermolyeva, "*Nezrimaya Armiya*" [The unseen army] in *Дочери России* [Daughters of Russia] (Russia, 1975).

2. P. M. H. Bell, *Twelve Turning Points of the Second World War* (New Haven, CT: Yale University Press, 2012), 98.

3. Ermolyeva, "*Nezrimaya Armiya*."

4. Ermolyeva, "*Nezrimaya Armiya*."

5. Ermolyeva, "*Nezrimaya Armiya*."

6. Ermolyeva, "*Nezrimaya Armiya*."

7. Sergey Medvedev, "Love and Penicillin," *Rostov City Journal*, November 1, 2014, https://kg-rostov.ru/history/histori_cult_person/lyubov-penitsillin/.

8. Medvedev, "Love and Penicillin."

9. Ermolyeva, "*Nezrimaya Armiya*."

10. Bell, *Twelve Turning Points*, 98.

11. Nina Chanishvili, *A Literature Review of the Practical Application of Bacteriophage Research* (Hauppauge, NY: Nova, 2012), chapter 3.

12. Chanishvili, *Literature Review*, chapter 3.

13. Chanishvili, *Literature Review*, chapter 3.

14. Chanishvili, *Literature Review*, chapter 3.

15. Nina Chanishvili, Dmitriy Myelnikov, and Timothy K. Blauvelt. "Professor Giorgi Eliava and the Eliava Institute of Bacteriophage," *Phage* 3, no. 2 (2022), https://doi.org/10.1089/phage.2022.0016.

16. Ermolyeva, "*Nezrimaya Armiya.*"

17. "Ermoleva, Zinaida (1898–1974)," Encyclopedia.com, https://www .encyclopedia.com/women/encyclopedias-almanacs-transcripts-and -maps/ermoleva-zinaida-1898-1974.

18. Ermolyeva, "*Nezrimaya Armiya.*"

19. Medvedev, "Love and Penicillin."

20. Medvedev, "Love and Penicillin."

21. Medvedev, "Love and Penicillin."

22. Medvedev, "Love and Penicillin."

23. Dmitriy Myelnikov, "An Alternative Cure: The Adoption and Survival of Bacteriophage Therapy in the USSR, 1922–1955," *Journal of the History of Medicine and Allied Sciences* 73, no. 4 (2018): 385–411, https:// doi.org/10.1093/jhmas/jry024.

24. Myelnikov, "An Alternative Cure."

25. Myelnikov, "An Alternative Cure."

26. Ermolyeva, "*Nezrimaya Armiya.*"

27. Ermolyeva, "*Nezrimaya Armiya.*"

28. Ermolyeva, "*Nezrimaya Armiya.*"

29. Myelnikov, "An Alternative Cure."

30. Myelnikov, "An Alternative Cure."

31. Myelnikov, "An Alternative Cure."

32. Myelnikov, "An Alternative Cure."

33. William C. Summers, *Félix d'Hérelle and the Origins of Molecular Biology* (New Haven, CT: Yale University Press, 1999), 48.

34. Monroe D. Eaton and Stanhope Bayne-Jones, "Bacteriophage Therapy: Review of the Principles and Results of the Use of Bacteriophage in the Treatment of Infections," *Journal of American Medical Association* 103, no. 23 (1934): 1769–76, https://doi.org/10.1001/ jama.1934.72750490003007.

35. William C. Summers, "The Strange History of Phage Therapy," *Bacteriophage* 2, no. 2 (2012): 130–3.

36. Summers, "The Strange History of Phage Therapy."

37. Myelnikov, "An Alternative Cure."

38. Dmitriy Myelnikov, "Creature Features: The Lively Narratives of Bacteriophages in Soviet Biology and Medicine," *The Royal Society Publishing* (2020), https://royalsocietypublishing.org/doi/10.1098 /rsnr.2019.0035.

8. The Rise of the Superbugs

1. Robert Fekety et al., "Staphylococcal Infections in the Hospital and Community," *American Journal of Public Health* 48, no. 3 (1958): 298–310, https://www.ncbi.nlm.nih.gov/pmc/articles/PMC1551528/.

2. Fekety et. al, "Staphylococcal Infections."

3. Fekety et. al, "Staphylococcal Infections."

4. R. T. Ravenholt and G. D. Laveck, "Staphylococcal Disease—An Obstetric, Pediatric, and Community Problem," *American Journal of Public Health* 46, no. 10 (1956): 1287–96, https://www.ncbi.nlm.nih.gov/pmc/articles/PMC1624081/.

5. Maryn McKenna, *Superbug: The Fatal Menace of MRSA* (New York: Free Press, 2010), 27.

6. Frank R. DeLeo et al., "Molecular Differentiation of Historic Phage-Type 80/81 and Contemporary Epidemic *Staphylococcus aureus*," *PNAS* 108, no. 44 (2011): 18091–6, https://www.pnas.org/doi/full/10.1073/pnas.1111084108.

7. Maryn McKenna, *Big Chicken: The Incredible Story of How Antibiotics Created Modern Agriculture and Changed the Way the World Eats* (Washington, DC: National Geographic, 2017), 45.

8. Thomas H. Jukes, "Some Historical Notes on Chlortetracycline," *Reviews of Infectious Diseases* 7, no. 5 (1985): 702–7, https://www.jstor.org/stable/4453725.

9. Jukes, "Some Historical Notes."

10. Jukes, "Some Historical Notes."

11. Jukes, "Some Historical Notes."

12. Jukes, "Some Historical Notes."

13. William L. Laurence, "'Wonder Drug' Aureomycin Found to Spur Growth 50%," *New York Times*, April 10, 1950, https://www.nytimes.com/1950/04/10/archives/wonder-drug-aureomycin-found-to-spur-growth-50-aureomycin-found.html.

14. Laurence, "'Wonder Drug.'"

15. E. Chain and E. Abraham, "An Enzyme from Bacteria Able to Destroy Penicillin," *Nature* 146 (1940): 837, https://doi.org/10.1038/146837a0.

16. Chain and Abraham, "An Enzyme from Bacteria."

17. D. Soufer, "Protecting Penicillin from Penicillinase," *Microbios* 45, no. 184–5 (1986): 193–8, https://pubmed.ncbi.nlm.nih.gov/3488490/#.

18. Alexander Fleming, "Penicillin," Nobel lecture, December 11, 1945, https://www.nobelprize.org/uploads/2018/06/fleming-lecture.pdf.

19. DeLeo et al., "Molecular Differentiation

20. McKenna, *Superbug*, 29–32.

21. DeLeo et al., "Molecular Differentiation."

22. DeLeo et al., "Molecular Differentiation."

23. C. L. Ventola, "The Antibiotic Resistance Crisis: Part 1: Causes and Threats," *Pharmacy and Therapeutics* 40, no. 4 (2015): 277–83, figure 1, https://www.ncbi.nlm.nih.gov/pmc/articles/PMC4378521/.

24. Ventola, "Antibiotic Resistance Crisis."

25. Ventola, "Antibiotic Resistance Crisis."

26. Ventola, "Antibiotic Resistance Crisis."

27. M. C. Enright et al., "The Evolutionary History of Methicillin-Resistant *Staphylococcus aureus* (MRSA)," *PNAS* 99, no. 11 (2002): 7687–92, https://doi.org/10.1073/pnas.122108599.

28. *Encyclopedia Britannica*, s.v. "Methicillin," https://www.britannica.com/science/methicillin.

29. Ventola, "Antibiotic Resistance Crisis."

30. David Shrayer-Petrov, *Staphylococcus Disease in the Soviet Union: Epidemiology and Response to a National Epidemic* (Falls Church, VA, Delphic Associates, Inc 1989), 25–6.

31. Shrayer-Petrov, *Staphylococcus Disease*, 25–6.

32. Shrayer-Petrov, *Staphylococcus Disease*, 25–6.

33. Shrayer-Petrov, *Staphylococcus Disease*, 25–6.

34. Nina Chanishvili, *A Literature Review of the Practical Application of Bacteriophage Research* (Hauppauge, NY: Nova, 2012), chapter 12.

35. Shrayer-Petrov, *Staphylococcus Disease*, 25–6; Anna Kuchment, *The Forgotten Cure: The Past and Future of Phage Therapy* (New York: Springer, 2012), 57.

36. Thomas Häusler, *Viruses vs. Superbugs: A Solution to the Antibiotic Crisis?* (London: Palgrave Macmillan, 2006), 172.

37. Häusler, *Viruses vs. Superbugs*, 172–3.

9. Phages Endangered

1. Nina Chanishvili, interview with the author, April 19, 2023.

2. Chanishvili interview, April 19, 2023.

3. Peter Radetsky, "The Good Virus," *Discover*, 1996, https://www

.discovermagazine.com/technology/the-good-virus; Chanishvili interview, April 19, 2023.

4. Chanishvili interview, April 19, 2023.
5. Mzia Kutateladze, interview with the author, April 15 and April 20, 2023.
6. Kutateladze interview, April 15 and April 20, 2023.
7. Radetsky, "The Good Virus."
8. Radetsky, "The Good Virus."

10. A Georgian in Maryland

1. Natela, Maia, and Mikhail Okudjava (Sandro's cousins), interview with the author, April 22, 2022.
2. Sandro Sulakvelidze, interview with the author, October 24, 2022.
3. Letters from Glenn Morris to the US embassy, June 1994, "Nino Visa Letters from Glenn-June 1994.pdf," Sandro Sulakvelidze family archives.
4. Letters from Morris to the US embassy.
5. Glenn Morris, interview with the author, December 20, 2021.
6. Morris interview, December 20, 2021.
7. Nina Chanishvili, interview with the author, April 22, 2023.
8. Chanishvili interview, April 22, 2023.
9. "Antibiotic Resistance - The Virus that Cures - BBC Horizon," YouTube video, 48:36, posted by Judith Bunting, June 27, 2020, https://www.youtube.com/watch?v=bmKMIP91lTE.
10. Richard Honour, interview with the author, October 23, 2023.
11. Richard Honour interview, October 23, 2023.
12. Richard Honour interview, October 23, 2023.
13. Richard Honour interview, October 23, 2023.
14. Richard Honour interview, October 23, 2023.
15. "Antibiotic Resistance," YouTube video.
16. Morris interview, December 20, 2021.
17. Sulakvelidze interview, October 24, 2022.
18. Sarah A. Egan et al., "Linezolid Resistance in *Enterococcus faecium* and *Enterococcus faecalis* from Hospitalized Patients in Ireland: High Prevalence of the MDR Genes *optrA* and *poxtA* in Isolates with Diverse Genetic Backgrounds," *Journal of Antimicrobial Chemotherapy* 75, no. 7 (2020): 1704–11, https://doi.org/10.1093/jac/dkaa075.

11. The Phage Whisperer

1. Biswajit Biswas, interview with the author, February 15, 2023.
2. Biswas interview, February 15, 2023.
3. Biswas interview, February 15, 2023.
4. J. Morison et al., "Cholera in a Khasi Village and Its Treatment with Bacteriophage," *The Indian Medical Gazette* 65, no. 3 (1930), https://www.ncbi.nlm.nih.gov/pmc/articles/PMC5157478/.
5. William C. Summers, *Félix d'Hérelle and the Origins of Molecular Biology* (New Haven, CT: Yale University Press, 1999), 125–44; Carl R. Merril, Dean Scholl, and Sankar L. Adhya, "The Prospect for Bacteriophage Therapy in Western Medicine," *Nature Reviews Drug Discovery* 2, no. 6 (2003): 489–97, https://doi.org/10.1038/nrd1111.
6. Biswas interview, February 15, 2023.
7. Carl Merril and Greg Merril, interview with the author, February 8, 2023.
8. Merril and Merril interview, February 8, 2023.
9. Merril and Merril interview, February 8, 2023.
10. Merril and Merril interview, February 8, 2023.
11. Biswas interview, February 15, 2023.
12. Biswas interview, February 15, 2023.
13. Biswas interview, February 15, 2023.
14. Biswas interview, February 15, 2023.
15. Merril and Merril interview, February 8, 2023.
16. Merril, Scholl, and Adhya, "The Prospect for Bacteriophage Therapy."
17. Merril and Merril interview, February 8, 2023.
18. Merril and Merril interview, February 8, 2023.

12. Naive and Stubborn, a Winning Combination

1. Sandro Sulakvelidze, interview with the author, October 24, 2022.
2. Sulakvelidze interview, October 24, 2022.
3. Carl Merril and Greg Merril, interview with the author, February 8, 2023.
4. Eric Boodman, "How the Navy Brought a Once-Derided Scientist Out of Retirement—And into the Virus-Selling Business," *STAT*, October 16, 2018, https://www.statnews.com/2018/10/16/phage-therapy-viruses-carl-merril-navy/.
5. Sandro Sulakvelidze, email with the author, January 2, 2024
6. Sulakvelidze interview, October 24, 2022.
7. Sandro Sulakvelidze, email with the author, November 22, 2022.

8. Sulakvelidze interview, October 24, 2022.

9. Steven Projan, "Phage-Inspired Antibiotics?," *Nature Biotechnology* 22, no. 2 (2004): 167–8, https://doi.org/10.1038/nbt0204-167.

10. Sulakvelidze interview, October 24, 2022.

11. Anna Kuchment, *The Forgotten Cure: The Past and Future of Phage Therapy* (New York: Springer, 2012), 101.

12. Sulakvelidze interview, October 24, 2022.

13. Sulakvelidze interview, October 24, 2022.

14. Sulakvelidze interview, October 24, 2022.

13. The Superbug That Won the Oscar—and the FDA

1. Steffanie Strathdee and Thomas Patterson, *The Perfect Predator: A Scientist's Race to Save Her Husband from a Deadly Superbug* (New York: Hachette, 2019), 175.

2. Strathdee and Patterson, *The Perfect Predator*, 71.

3. Ryland Young, interview with the author, May 21, 2023.

4. Young interview, May 21, 2023.

5. M. Liu et al., "Comparative Genomics of *Acinetobacter baumannii* and Therapeutic Bacteriophages from a Patient Undergoing Phage Therapy," *Nature Communications* 13, no. 1 (2022): 3776, https://doi .org/10.1038/s41467-022-31455-5.

6. Strathdee and Patterson, *The Perfect Predator*, 96.

7. Maya Merabishvili et al., "Characterization of newly isolated lytic bacteriophages active against Acinetobacter baumannii," *PLOS One* (2014): e104853, https://journals.plos.org/plosone/arti cle?id=10.1371/journal.pone.0104853.

8. Robert "Chip" Schooley, interview with the author, April 13, 2022.

9. Strathdee and Patterson, *The Perfect Predator*, 145–6.

10. Strathdee and Patterson, *The Perfect Predator*, 167.

11. Young interview, May 21, 2023.

12. Young interview, May 21, 2023.

13. Young interview, May 21, 2023.

14. Young interview, May 21, 2023.

15. Schooley interview, April 13, 2022.

16. National Institutes of Health, *Facing the Reality of Drug-Resistant Tuberculosis in India: Challenges and Potential Solutions: Summary of a Joint Workshop by the Institute of Medicine, the Indian National Science Academy, and the Indian Council of Medical Research* (Washington,

DC: National Academies Press, 2012), https://www.ncbi.nlm.nih.gov
/books/NBK100386/.

17. Rodrigo E. Mendes et al., "Longitudinal (2001–14) Analysis of
Enterococci and VRE Causing Invasive Infections in European and US
Hospitals, Including a Contemporary (2010–13) Analysis of Orita-
vancin *in vitro* Potency," *Journal of Antimicrobial Chemotherapy* 71, no.
12 (2016): 3453–8, https://doi.org/10.1093/jac/dkw319.

18. E. S. Snitkin et al., "Tracking a Hospital Outbreak of Carbapenem-
Resistant *Klebsiella pneumoniae* with Whole-Genome Sequencing,"
Science Translational Medicine 4, no. 148 (2012): 148ra116, https://doi
.org/10.1126/scitranslmed.3004129.

19. *Antibiotic Resistance Threats in the United States, 2013* (Atlanta, GA:
CDC, 2013), https://www.cdc.gov/drugresistance/pdf/ar-threats
-2013-508.pdf.

20. Cara Fiore, interview with the author, March 3, 2023.

21. Schooley interview, April 13, 2022.

22. Schooley interview, April 13, 2022.

23. Young interview, May 21, 2023.

24. Carl Merril and Greg Merril, interview with the author, February 8,
2023.

25. Biswajit Biswas, interview with the author, February 15, 2023.

26. Merril and Merril interview, February 8, 2023.

27. Biswajit Biswas interview, February 15, 2023.

28. Merril and Merril interview, February 8, 2023.

29. Merril and Merril interview, February 8, 2023.

30. Merril and Merril interview, February 8, 2023.

31. Theron Hamilton, interview with the author, June 20, 2023.

32. Young interview, May 21, 2023.

33. Strathdee and Patterson, *The Perfect Predator,* 229.

34. Merril and Merril interview, February 8, 2023.

35. Strathdee and Patterson, *The Perfect Predator*, 274–5.

36. Strathdee and Patterson, *The Perfect Predator*, 269.

14. The Perfect Storm's Aftermath

1. Sandro Sulakvelidze, interview with the author, February 28, 2023.

2. Sulakvelidze interview, February 28, 2023.

3. "Groundbreaking Study Led by the Crohn's & Colitis Foundation Estimates Nearly 1 in 100 Americans Has Inflammatory Bowel Disease

(IBD)," Crohn's & Colitis Foundation, July 20, 2023, https://www
.crohnscolitisfoundation.org/groundbreaking-study-led-the-crohns
-colitis-foundation-estimates-nearly-1-100-americans-has.

4. Maiko Sasaki et al., "Invasive *Escherichia coli* Are a Feature of Crohn's
   Disease," *Laboratory Investigation* 87 (2007): 1042–54, https://www
   .nature.com/articles/3700661.

5. Sasaki et al., "Invasive *Escherichia coli*."

6. Sulakvelidze interview, February 28, 2023.

7. *Antibiotic Resistance Threats in the United States, 2013* (Atlanta, GA:
   CDC, 2013), https://www.cdc.gov/drugresistance/pdf/ar-threats
   -2013-508.pdf.

8. C. L. Ventola, "The Antibiotic Resistance Crisis: Part 1: Causes and
   Threats," *Pharmacy and Therapeutics* 40, no. 4 (2015): 277–83, https:
   //www.ncbi.nlm.nih.gov/pmc/articles/PMC4378521/.

9. Joseph Campbell, interview with the author, December 20, 2022.

10. Robert "Chip" Schooley, interview with the author, April 13, 2022.

11. Cara Fiore, interview with the author, March 3, 2023.

12. Fiore interview, March 3, 2023.

13. Saima Aslam et al., "Lessons Learned from the First 10 Consecutive
    Cases of Intravenous Bacteriophage Therapy to Treat Multidrug-
    Resistant Bacterial Infections at a Single Center in the United States,"
    Open Forum Infectious Diseases 7, no. 9 (2020): ofaa389, https://www
    .ncbi.nlm.nih.gov/pmc/articles/PMC7519779/.

14. Paul Garofolo, interview with the author, May 1, 2023.

15. Graham Hatfull, interview with the author, April 17, 2023.

16. R. M. Dedrick et al., "Engineered Bacteriophages for Treatment of a
    Patient with a Disseminated Drug-Resistant *Mycobacterium abscessus*,"
    Nature Medicine 25 (2019): 730–3, https://www.nature.com/arti
    cles/s41591-019-0437-z.

17. Dedrick et al., "Engineered Bacteriophages."

18. Hatfull interview, April 17, 2023.

19. John O'Halloran, "Total Joint Replacement: Statistics for Post-
    Surgery and Rehabilitation," MedBridge, May 18, 2022, https://www
    .medbridge.com/blog/2022/05/total-joint-replacement-statistics-for
    -post-surgery-and-rehabilitation/.

20. John and Barbara Haverty, interview with the author, April 11 and
    May 20, 2023.

21. Gina Suh, interview with the author, April 28, 2023.

22. Suh interview, April 28, 2023.

23. Suh interview, April 28, 2023.

24. Daniel Moskalenko, interview with the author, August 30, 2023.

25. Andrey and Anya Zvyagintsev, interview with the author, August 28, 2023.

26. William C. Summers, *Félix d'Hérelle and the Origins of Molecular Biology* (New Haven, CT: Yale University Press, 1999), 126.

27. "Buruli Ulcer, a Neglected Disease," Epicentre, updated February 21, 2022, https://epicentre.msf.org/en/portfolio/buruli-ulcer.

28. Tobi Nagel, interview with the author, May 26, 2023.

15. Phaging into the Future

1. Mzia Kutateladze, interview with the author, April 20, 2022.

2. Vakhtang Pavlenishvili, interview with the author, April 20, 2022.

3. Steffanie Strathdee, interview with the author on Oct 31, 2022.

4. Strathdee interview Oct 31, 2022.

5. Paul Garofolo, interview with the author on May 1, 2023.

6. Cara Fiore, interview with the author, March 3, 2023; E. Scott Stibitz, interview with the author, March 3, 2023.

INDEX

ABOUT THE AUTHOR

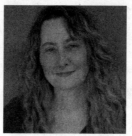

Mallory Pettee

Lina Zeldovich grew up in a dissident family of Soviet scientists and learned English as a second language in her twenties as an immigrant New Yorker. Now an award-winning journalist, author, speaker, and Columbia Journalism School alumna, she has contributed hundreds of stories for leading publications, which include *Popular Science, The New York Times, Reader's Digest, Scientific American, Smithsonian, National Geographic,* and *BBC Future,* and has appeared on radio, podcasts, and television. Zeldovich is the author of *The Other Dark Matter: The Science and Business of Turning Waste into Wealth and Health.* She lives in New York City.